"Unlike any other book I have read on this subject, *Not Your Mother's Hysterectomy* reads more like a memoir than a medical reference. It touches your heart, educates your mind, and compels you to take a journey through the eyes of a surgeon and her patients . . . all women who are facing a fight with cancer or other serious medical illnesses together."

RANDY FAGIN, MD
CHIEF ADMINISTRATIVE OFFICER, THE TEXAS INSTITUTE FOR ROBOTIC SURGERY
SENIOR MEDICAL ADVISOR FOR US TRAINING, INTUITIVE SURGICAL

"I am one of those women whose mother had a bad experience with her hysterectomy. I can personally attest to the fact that times have changed. Dr. Kowalski is a professional who listens and truly cares about women's health. Her book provides honest information to help guide women through the surgery and better understand that today, we, as patients, are an integral part of the decisions that affect our health and our lives."

BARBARA K. CEGAVSKE
NEVADA STATE SENATOR
SENATE HUMAN RESOURCES, VICE CHAIR
MEMBER, NEVADA STATE LEGISLATIVE COMMITTEE ON HEALTH CARE

"Dr Kowalski has always impressed me as an outstanding surgeon but also as a person. Her enthusiasm for education and advancement of surgical techniques is once more demonstrated in this book. It provides an easy-to-read description and understanding of common gynecological conditions, both benign and malignant, with real patient stories. She provides practical and valuable information on the advancements of hysterectomy technology, and particularly the robotic approach of which she has been a pioneer."

DR. JAVIER MAGRINA
DIRECTOR, GYNECOLOGIC ONCOLOGY
PROFESSOR OF OBGYN, MAYO GRADUATE SCHOOL OF MEDICINE
BARBARA WOODWARD LIPS PROFESSOR

D0839286

"As the daughter of an obstetrician/gynecologist, I was schooled early in life about the joys of being a female. I was always urged to take full responsibility for my own good health, to listen to my body and take care of it as if it were made of the finest fabric. I was to learn, to ask questions and to respect what was right for my own health. If and when problems might arise, I was told always to 'explore your options, never leave anything to chance or potential serious problems to just one opinion.' So here I am these many years later having lived so well by that dictum and having imparted the same clear message to all of my children (three boys and a girl). I am delighted to read that Dr. Kowalski is the strongest advocate for pursuing the best opportunities for a lifetime of good health."

CAROLYN G. GOODMAN
MAYOR, CITY OF LAS VEGAS

"This book provides a lot of reassurance for women who are facing a hysterectomy. It takes away a lot of the mystery and explains how surgeons think and also talks about all of the options. I think any woman or her family that is facing a hysterectomy would find this book extremely valuable."

BARBARA GOFF, MD
DIRECTOR, GYNECOLOGIC ONCOLOGY
UNIVERSITY OF WASHINGTON AND SEATTLE CANCER CARE ALLIANCE

N T
Y UR
M THER'S
HYSTERECT MY

*A Transformation
in Women's Health Care*

LYNN D. KOWALSKI, MD

Publisher	*Corey Michael Blake*
Executive Editor	*Katie Gutierrez*
Staff Editor	*Pamela DeLoatch*
Creative Director	*David Charles Cohen*
Directoress of Happiness	*Erin Cohen*
Director of Author Services	*Kristin Westberg*
Facts Keeper	*Mike Winicour*
Cover Design	*Analee Paz*
Print and Digital Interior Design	*Sunny DiMartino*
Proofreading	*Rita Hess*
Last Looks	*Sunny DiMartino*
Print and Digital Post Production	*Sunny DiMartino*

Writers of the Round Table Press
PO Box 511, Highland Park, IL 60035
www.roundtablecompanies.com

Printed in the United States of America
First Edition: December 2013
10 9 8 7 6 5 4 3 2 1

Library of Congress Cataloging-in-Publication Data
Kowalksi, Lynn D.
Not your mother's hysterectomy: a transformation in women's health care /
Lynn D. Kowalski.—1st ed. p. cm.
ISBN Paperback   978-1-939418-48-7
ISBN Digital   978-1-939418-49-4
Library of Congress Control Number   2013954884

RTC Publishing is an imprint of Writers of the Round Table, Inc. Writers of the Round Table Press and the RTC Publishing logo are trademarks of Writers of the Round Table, Inc.

The information provided in this book is designed to provide helpful information on the subjects discussed. This book is not meant to be used, nor should it be used, to diagnose or treat any medical condition. For diagnosis or treatment of any medical problem, consult your own physician. The publisher and author are not responsible for any specific health or allergy needs that may require medical supervision and are not liable for any damages or negative consequences from any treatment, action, application, or preparation, to any person reading or following the information in this book. References are provided for informational purposes only and do not constitute endorsement of any medical procedures, treatments, websites, or other sources. Readers should be aware that the websites listed in this book may change.

TABLE OF CONTENTS

ACKNOWLEDGMENTS

I would like to thank the many people who helped me with this book. First, for the inspiration to let the idea for this book take shape, I would like to thank my friend Barbara Cegavske. Her experience with her mother's health care showed me a real need for this project. Devin Hughes was instrumental in connecting me to RTC publishers who could make my work a reality.

I am grateful to my aunt, Laura Buss, for providing insight and editing advice along the way. To my editors Katie Gutierrez and Pamela DeLoatch, who must now feel they know more about gynecology, female anatomy, and women's health than they ever thought possible, thank you for all your hard work and for bringing out the best in me. To Corey Blake, thank you for believing in this project and allowing me to see it to its fruition.

To Drs. Javier Magrina, John Boggess, and Randy Fagin, pioneers in robotic surgery, thank you for sharing your innovative spirit and expertise. I am also forever grateful to Billy Trengove, the Intuitive Surgical rep whose persistence and charm got me to take him seriously.

To my lifetime and business partner, Stephanie Wishnev, thank you for being with me through the good times and the bad, and for supporting and encouraging me through this project from start to finish. You have helped make me the best doctor I can be.

To Roni Lowery, Joyce Reed, Dara Marias, and all the patients who have put their confidence in me over my years of practice, I am forever grateful for the opportunity to be your doctor. Your trust in me is what makes it all worthwhile.

For Stephanie

My Gold Standard

FOREWORD *by* DARA MARIAS

By the time I was 36 years old, I had lost my mother, aunt, and grandmother to cancer. My grandmother had bilateral breast cancer and stomach cancer. My mother had ovarian cancer and breast cancer. Her half-sister died of breast cancer before I was born. There was a good bet that this was not by chance and that our family had a genetic mutation responsible for these cancers.

About three months after my grandmother passed away, I realized that it was time for me to confront my genetic make-up. I walked into the lab, gave one vial of blood, and walked out. A weight had been lifted—I would finally find out if I had the suspected "BRCA" mutation that would confer an 87 percent lifetime risk of breast cancer and a 40 to 60 percent risk of ovarian cancer. I had a 50/50 chance.

A few weeks later, I had my answer: I was BRCA positive. From the minute I received the results, I knew one thing for sure: I would take action and remove those parts of my body that were susceptible to hereditary cancer. This meant prophylactic or "preventative" surgeries to remove my uterus, fallopian tubes, ovaries, and breast tissue. I had decided well in advance that if the results came back positive, I would do everything in my power to ensure that my outcome would be different than that of my mother and family. The enormity of the road that lay ahead of me, however, was daunting. Where to begin?

My situation was complicated by the fact that I had a complete and utter fear of surgery. I hadn't always felt that way. My view of doctors and surgeons was dramatically colored by my mother's experience during treatment of her ovarian cancer. After my mom underwent chemotherapy, she had a laparoscopic procedure to biopsy her abdomen and make sure her cancer was gone. During this procedure, however, the surgeon (not Dr. Kowalski) accidentally cut into her bowel in several places, causing my mother to become septic. Within a week of her surgery, my mother was in a coma in ICU. She remained there for three and a half months, followed by another three months in Intermediate Care. She underwent more than 20 additional surgeries and was left with gaping holes in her abdomen that took more than a year to close. She was never the same. It was horrific, and the images of her experience were seared in my mind.

After my mother's experience, I was, in short order, petrified to undergo surgery on my abdomen; yet, I clearly needed to. Dr. Kowalski had been my doctor for a few years at the time I went to her office to share the results. We both knew what I needed to do, and we both knew my feelings about surgery. Part of the issue with my mom's surgery was the extensive scarring in her abdomen from the prior ovarian cancer surgery and the limitations of the laparoscopic procedure. Having had two prior C-sections, I was certain that my scar tissue would be an issue for me, too. Under no circumstances was I going to have a laparoscopic procedure. Dr. Kowalski knew me, knew my mom, and respectfully agreed to perform the old-fashioned "Gold Standard" surgery. This would involve a large, vertical midline incision and was major abdominal surgery with extended recovery. But this was what I wanted, because I was afraid of a laparoscopic procedure.

One day, about three weeks before my surgery, I was scheduled to see Dr. Kowalski. Just before I left, my husband, often the voice of reason in my life, asked me if I had ever sat down with Dr. Kowalski to explore other, less invasive, options. He pointed out the risks of the major surgery I was contemplating and then gave me an important piece of advice. He said, "If you trust Dr. Kowalski implicitly, shouldn't you trust her to advise you what is right?" He pointed out that my choice of the "Big Cut" was born of fear, not counsel from my doctor.

That day, I asked Dr. Kowalski about it: "Given my circumstances, not my mother's, what would you advise for me?"

I half expected her to recommend a laparoscopic hysterectomy. Instead, her response was out of left field. "You would be a perfect candidate for robotic-assisted laparoscopic surgery."

My first thought was, *Did she just say robots?*

Once I got over my shock, Dr. Kowalski began to explain the da Vinci hysterectomy to me. By the time she was done, it was like a whole new world had opened up. My fear of the surgeon not having a clear enough view was completed assuaged by the knowledge that by using the da Vinci Surgical System, Dr. Kowalski would have a *better* view than in open surgery. She would see in high definition and 10-times magnification using the da Vinci equipment. I discovered that there was minimal blood loss, a faster healing time, and an overall much easier recuperation. As fearful as I was of surgery, I knew that what she was saying was right for me and my circumstances. After all, Dr. Kowalski was the same person who had taken time to painstakingly answer every question I had about the procedure and what organs to remove, and she had even analyzed various studies about hormone replacement with me. She had always been my partner in this process, and as I left her office, I realized that through her guidance and sensitivity, she had empowered me to finally make an informed and logical choice.

My hysterectomy experience ended up being a blip on the radar of my life. Despite the significance of the procedure, the recovery was amazingly fast. My two C-sections were a much harder recuperation. I felt like I had a few cuts on my stomach. I simply could not believe how easy it was in comparison.

I share my story not to suggest that minimally invasive surgery is right for everyone and every circumstance. Rather, my point is that I would have never had this outcome had I not asked the right questions and had the right doctor. Whether you come to your hysterectomy because of fibroids, endometriosis, BRCA mutations, cancer, or any other reason—the single most important factor in making the right decisions for *you* is becoming an educated patient. I made sure I knew everything there was to know about the procedures I would undergo and the diagnosis I received. There simply is no substitute for an honest and educated exchange with your doctor.

Not Your Mother's Hysterectomy: A Transformation in Women's Health Care has all of the information you need to be your own advocate. Through this book, Dr. Kowalski will do for you what she did for me—she will demystify the hysterectomy process and empower you to make the choices that are right for you in your situation. While the book can be read front to back, Dr. Kowalski has also made the information easily accessible by topic. If you have heard a term or procedure in any way related to a hysterectomy, it will be in this book.

In addition, Dr. Kowalski takes complicated medical procedures and jargon and breaks them down to make them understandable— even to those of us without medical degrees! She explains in detail every aspect of the procedures, including how to prepare for the surgery and what to expect after the surgery in the days and weeks to come. What I especially appreciated about the book are the examples of real patients interspersed throughout. More likely than not, you will identify with one of the women whose stories are profiled by Dr. Kowalski. In these stories, Dr. Kowalski provides insight into how she approached care in these varying health scenarios. Irrespective of your doctor's approach, this knowledge gives you a starting point for conversation. Taken together with "Questions for My Surgeon," you will be well on your way to ensuring that you work with a doctor with whom you have trust and rapport.

Finally, in writing this book, Dr. Kowalski bravely shares her own experiences facing and overcoming large life obstacles. Like those of us whose health has forced us on a path we would not have chosen, Dr. Kowalski knows what it feels like to confront such obstacles and move forward to a better tomorrow. Life is about personal transformation, and I believe that the information provided in this book will empower and transform you into your own best advocate, ultimately allowing you to move forward from this difficult time and evolve into a new, healthier you!

Dara Marias, Esquire

PREFACE

"You need a hysterectomy."

Few words are as alarming for a woman to hear. Not only is there the dread of the actual operation and recovery, but there's also the fear of the condition that necessitated it. But perhaps most chilling is that this particular operation, which removes the reproductive organs, strikes at the very core of our femininity.

I'm a woman—a woman who is also a surgeon. As a female surgeon who cares for female patients, I know that one of the uniquely female experiences in life is the prospect of a hysterectomy. Nearly one-third of all American women will undergo this operation during their lifetime. Whether you need a hysterectomy for abnormal bleeding, for pain, or for cancer, it's scary to face major surgery. Will you feel better afterward? Will you still feel like a woman? How long will it take to recover? How risky is a hysterectomy? Although it's natural to ask family or friends who went through one how it turned out for them, sometimes their stories can make you feel even more apprehensive. Your mom's recovery seemed so difficult. Why did your aunt need such a big incision? Who was your neighbor's doctor? He never explained anything to her. Some of the complications sound horrendous. But times have changed, and modern approaches can make it easier than you might expect. The hysterectomy of today is not the hysterectomy of your mother's or grandmother's era.

As a gynecologic oncologist, I specialize in the care of women needing hysterectomies for all kinds of problems, including cancer. I have taken care of thousands of women facing an operation that can feel like a turning point in their lives. In the early days of my training, I saw one woman after another suffer through the emotional and physical toll of a difficult surgical recovery. The operations seemed so invasive, so disfiguring. Large incisions from the belly button to the pubic bone were the norm, and some incisions were even longer. It seemed as though medicine was stuck in an old way of approaching such a common female experience. Women undergoing these surgeries seemed disembodied from the process, as if the operation was done *to* them, not *with* them. I was complicit in this old-fashioned mindset, partly from being stuck in the old medical paradigm and partly from my own immaturity. However, in 2005, I went through a personal experience that helped change my whole approach to surgery and to my patients. My practice transformed, and so did my patients' experience of the hysterectomy process. Now, I see women who feel surprised at how much easier the surgery was than they expected.

I wrote this book to share this transformation with you. I use real stories of women I have taken care of in my practice. For privacy reasons, I have used fake names for most cases. The details of each case, though, are real and are meant to help you through your own journey. If you see yourself in some of my patients, it's because many women face similar circumstances. However, every woman is unique. Do not mistake a recommendation for one of my own patients as medical advice directed to you. Always seek the advice of your own doctor when deciding how to approach your health care. The information in this book is for educational purposes only and can never substitute for a personal examination and discussion with your own physician.

Because of my personal bias, I will avoid the cumbersome generic pronoun "he/she" when referring to surgeons and just call all surgeons "she." I do this with the acknowledgement that many surgeons are men, but, as I write this book from my own experience, I am clearly giving you my perspective as a woman surgeon. Imagining myself in the operating room as we go through this book, the pronoun "she" seems most appropriate.

I would also like to clarify that I work in a private practice setting, and I am not employed by any surgical company. As you will learn from reading this book, I have a strong bias toward less invasive surgical techniques. In particular, I recommend robotic surgery whenever possible. The surgical robot is a computer interface between surgeon and patient that allows complex operations to be performed through tiny incisions. The brand most widely used is manufactured by Intuitive Surgical Inc., a company based in Sunnyvale, California. I do not own stock in the company, nor do I work for them. Over the years, I have done some consulting work for the company and have taught other surgeons how to perform robotic surgery. I do not make more money doing robotic surgery. Neither Medicare nor private insurance companies recognize robotic surgery as a unique method of hysterectomy, so there is no additional payment for doing the surgery this way.

We live in an information age, where we have nearly instant access to vast resources of knowledge. As a result, we usually look things up on the Internet before making choices about many important decisions. For example, we can go buy a car armed with a full report of the dealer's costs, the available options, and financing packages. We can search for a new home mortgage on the Internet, comparing the different interest rates, terms, and penalties. We *participate* in the process, rather than just passively going along for the ride. We make our voices heard, rather than just accepting the status quo. We seek expertise, and then we make choices.

But what about our health care? Our interactions with the medical system remain, in many cases, archaic. As it has been for decades, we go to the doctor vulnerable and naïve. We don't know enough to know better, so we don't understand the options available to us. Unless you've gone to medical school, medical science is a daunting subject. Medical technology is progressing at breakneck speed with more complicated treatments available all the time. How do you become a *participant* in your health care, rather than just a recipient of it? Through education. That is what I hope this book gives you.

Your empowerment elevates a new generation of women.

Chapter 1

MY JOURNEY WITH ROBOTIC SURGERY

In early 2005, my life took an unexpected turn that would change me forever.

In a matter of days, everything I thought I knew about my practice and the people I worked with was shattered. Although there were hints of problems, there was no way to prepare for the scale of the meltdown that occurred.

At the time, I belonged to a large group of specialty surgeons with many offices spanning two states. In 1998, one of the senior partners recruited me right out of my surgical training in gynecologic oncology. Back then, I was naïve and trusting. (Unfortunately, they don't teach business sense in medical school.) After only a few years with the group, I was proud to make partner.

Then something went very wrong: without warning, the doctors at one of the locations were evicted from their office because the rent hadn't been paid in months. The partners held an emergency meeting. Those of us who lived out-of-state from the group headquarters, including me, flew in. We were unceremoniously informed that the practice was bankrupt. We had all worked hard and carried extremely busy practices, but it didn't matter: there was no money to pay our salaries or, worse, our bills.

At this meeting, the harsh reality of our situation was laid out before us. Millions of dollars were missing. We had to vote on whether to remove the head of the group from his managerial position. I listened to the information presented to us and voted with the majority—to remove him. But there was not unanimity. Factions developed among the partners.

When I returned home, the doctor who had just been voted out called me. "I'm moving in, and I'm going to run you out of town," he threatened.

His words scared me, but they also made me determined to prove him wrong. By March, about six weeks into this mess, he had moved in.

At the time all this was happening, the senior partner was on medical leave for a knee replacement, and I was covering our practice on my own. He had sided with the minority, on the side of the managing partner. Within a week of the senior partner returning to work, I saw him across the nursing station while I was making rounds on the hospital ward. He sat within earshot of me, and I heard him proudly tell another doctor, "Well, the first thing I did when I got back from my surgery was to get rid of Kowalski."

I thought, *He didn't get rid of me. I'm still here and still a partner in this group.*

But the writing was on the wall and I realized I needed to find a new office. I began making plans to lease a space from some colleagues. On April 1, a Friday, I went to my old office with a car full of cardboard boxes and a few helpers to collect my patient charts and my personal belongings. I needed the charts to continue caring for my cancer patients.

A burly bodyguard with a gun on his belt greeted me at the door. When I explained that I was there to move my belongings and my charts, he threatened me. First verbally. Then he grabbed me, wrapping his meaty hand around my upper arm and shoving me toward the door. His grip was so tight, I thought if I struggled or tried to wrench away, he would break my arm. The office staff, people I had worked with for seven years, watched idly as the threat escalated. I cast my gaze around at them, looking for anyone to step in and help, but they each looked away.

Empty handed, I stood in the lobby of my office building looking at the door as it closed in my face. I had worked unthinkably long hours, sacrificed my youth and my relationships to devote myself to medicine and to my patients. And now, it was all gone: my belongings, my charts, and my practice were on the other side of that door. I held back the tears—but just barely.

I went out to my car, parked in the hot desert sun, and sat there in disbelief. The smell of warm cardboard from the unused boxes stung my nostrils. I felt burned, humiliated, and angry. I opened the windows, took a few deep breaths, and started making phone calls, desperate for someone to help me recover what I had lost. Then I started moving forward, just focusing on getting things done. I finished preparing the temporary office over the weekend and started seeing patients that Monday.

I had no employees, no charts, not a stick of furniture, no business knowledge, and no money. I only had phone numbers for a few patients because I had managed to spirit my appointment book out of the old office. My mother-in-law stepped in, offering to act as receptionist for patients I prayed would come.

I had been through many difficulties before in my life, starting with my parents' divorce when I was five and including a grueling medical school and residency experience, but this . . . this was my lowest point. Even though it seemed as if I was surviving the catastrophe, putting the pieces of my new practice in place, I still felt shaken loose from my foundation. I didn't know what crisis would occur next, what demanding phone calls I would get about my previous group, what roadblocks I'd soon encounter. After weeks of stress, the constant tension was taking its toll on me. I didn't sleep. I felt disillusioned with people, disheartened with medicine, and angry with myself for getting involved in such a sordid situation. Why hadn't I seen the red flags as easily as I would have noticed a patient's symptoms? I had always been a naturally trusting person, and now I looked down on myself for that quality. This was not at all what I had envisioned when I decided, at the age of five, that I wanted to be a doctor.

Ironically, that dream was born the same day my parents' divorce decree was signed. It had been a long, weary process that dragged on for months. Mom was just coming home from court. I was watching a kids' game show on television, jumping up and down on the couch as I encouraged one kid to win. When he did, I was so excited that I jumped extra high and slipped on the couch on the way down. My cheek collided with the edge of the coffee table, and Mom walked in to find me on the floor with a cut on the side of my face and blood everywhere.

She grabbed a towel to staunch the blood and rushed me to our local family doctor. He spoke gently and confidently to me.

"You're going to need a few stitches, but everything will be okay."

He made me feel so calm that I didn't even flinch when he put the numbing needle in my cheek. My mother held my hand firmly, and I felt brave. We would get through this together. I could feel the stitches going through my skin, but it didn't hurt. The smell of antiseptic and all those clean glass jars filled with cotton balls comforted me. In that moment, I knew I wanted to be a doctor.

Thirty-five years later, my reputation as a good doctor saved me from financial ruin. I had to pick up the pieces and claw my way back to some semblance of normalcy. Many of my patients followed me to my temporary location until I could get on my feet again. Doctors in my community continued to refer patients to me. But the deeper wounds were still there.

As it turns out, though, something great also happened in April of 2005. The FDA approved the *da Vinci*® Surgical System for use in gynecology. By September, my new practice was thriving, but I was still dealing with the ongoing legal quagmire of the ugly breakup. One day in the hospital, I was approached by Billy Trengove, a salesperson from the company that manufactures *da Vinci*. His job was to introduce this new technology to accomplished surgeons who might appreciate its benefits. He had heard about my surgical skills and my strong interest in minimally invasive surgery. Doctors are approached by pharmacy and medical instrumentation salespeople all the time, and sometimes we tune them out, but eventually, what he said got my attention.

"Dr. Kowalski, I think you would be an ideal fit for this technology and the benefits it offers," he began, as handsome and charming as most pharmaceutical sales reps are. "It's just been approved for gynecological surgery, and there are only a few people in the country using it so far. You could be one of the first."

We sat down in the doctor's lounge and, over bad hospital food, we discussed some of my frustrations with the current state of gynecologic surgery.

"So what can robotic surgery do for me?" I challenged him. But a little voice in my head told me I was actually challenging myself. I already felt that I had maximized my potential using the surgical techniques available at the time. I had seen firsthand the enormous gap between healing from an old-fashioned hysterectomy (known as the "Big Cut") and the newer approaches (a few dime-sized incisions). Women from previous generations suffered from the pain, loss of independence, and scarring from open surgery. The laparoscopic hysterectomy of 2005 couldn't be done for more complicated cases, but these were the women who needed it most; the more complicated the case, the greater the benefit from less invasive surgery.

As we talked, I felt a stir of excitement that had been missing for months—perhaps years. Given what I had recently been through, I was eager to learn something new that would bridge this gap and renew my joy in medicine. I expected to learn a new tool. I never dreamed I was on the cusp of a surgical revolution.

"Name three areas in your practice where you'd like to offer the benefits of minimally invasive surgery to more women," Billy said.

The answers were easy.

"Radical hysterectomy for cervical cancer," I said, ticking it off my finger. This operation for early cervical cancer defines the skill and training of a gynecologic oncologist. Traditionally, women underwent a radical hysterectomy through an open incision with a prolonged and difficult recovery. At that time, some surgeons had reported their experience trying to perform the operation laparoscopically, but most gynecologic oncologists were reluctant to adopt this approach. Many felt unable to perform the steps of this cancer operation satisfactorily due to the inherent limitations of conventional laparoscopy. Lack of vision and reduced dexterity are compounded in such a complex operation. But many surgeons felt torn because minimally invasive surgery would be such a huge benefit to cancer patients! After years of watching women suffer through the long recovery of the old-fashioned radical hysterectomy, I dreamed of finding a better way.

"Second, operating on obese patients," I said as Billy nodded and jotted notes on a yellow pad. These cases really challenge a surgeon's skills, persistence, and confidence. Obese patients can benefit most from minimally invasive surgery due to the host of problems associated with big open incisions. But in many cases, standard hysterectomy approaches like a conventional laparoscopic hysterectomy are technically impossible in the obese, especially the severely obese. Although I wanted to avoid large incisions as much as possible, there was no viable alternative.

"And third, patients who have had extensive previous surgery," I said.

Historically, previous operations meant a hysterectomy must be done through an open incision because of the risk of scar tissue. These patients were almost always denied the opportunity to enjoy the benefits of minimally invasive surgery. The logic said all that scar tissue required advanced surgical dexterity and could not be dealt with safely using conventional laparoscopy.

After exploring the challenges on my list, Billy asked me to come and watch one case. As interesting as this sounded, I was still rebuilding my practice and was reluctant to travel.

"Dr. Kowalski, the challenges you've described are the very problems the *da Vinci* was designed to solve. Can you risk not seeing it?" Billy asked.

I gave in and agreed to a trip to the Mayo Clinic for a case observation. I had the good fortune to meet and learn from one of the great surgical masters of my field, Dr. Javier Magrina. He was genuine and welcoming, a dark-haired, handsome man from Spain. A natural teacher and real gentleman, he talked as he operated, showcasing an elegant style that immediately appealed to me. People don't realize that surgery is an intensely physical act, and many surgeons find their careers shortened by neck, shoulder, and back problems. If old-fashioned laparoscopy resembled a first-time runner slogging through the last mile of a marathon, Dr. Magrina was dancing a fine ballet. I watched him perform a hysterectomy with no blood loss and minimal tissue trauma, and I knew I was looking at the future of surgery.

That night, I dreamt about surgery for the first time in many years. In the dream, I was in an operating room with a patient, sitting in a special chair with some type of headset on. I was thinking the steps of the operation. I thought, *Grasp here and move to the left*, and it grasped and moved to the left. I thought, *Coagulate the blood vessels here*, and it did. I was literally thinking the operation into reality! When I woke up, I knew my dream was still in the realm of science fiction, but the idea of a better way to operate was burned in my brain, and I was determined to make it so.

I quickly attended a hands-on laboratory and spent hours practicing with the new technology. Looking forward to my first case, I was a newbie all over again. It was important to find the right type of case: one that would be simple for someone learning a new technique. I found a patient who was a good candidate—a very straightforward case that I would normally have performed with a conventional laparoscopic hysterectomy. I explained the new technology to her and asked her permission to be my first case. She agreed and was the first patient in the state of Nevada to have a robotic hysterectomy. The operation went well, but I was slower than usual and not very elegant. It was challenging, sobering, for an accomplished surgeon to feel like an intern again. With laparoscopic surgery, there's added pressure, because everyone in the room can see exactly what the surgeon is doing on big-screen monitors. Afterward, however, my patient's quick recovery amazed me. I was not expecting such a difference compared to conventional laparoscopic surgery.

I began discussing the technique with other patients and gaining additional experience with more straightforward cases. Eventually, I felt confident enough to offer robotic surgery to the patients who needed it most—the ones on my list with the challenges I had struggled with for so long. By case 42, I performed my first robotic radical hysterectomy. Wow! What a difference! I could see everything so much clearer—the tiny blood vessels, the lymph nodes, the ureters. I was satisfied with the quality of the surgery, and the patient's recovery was a breeze. I thought back to my training days, when the hospital ward was full of women with huge incisions lying in their beds in pain. This patient went home the next day and was back to yoga after a month.

Over the years, robotic surgery has transformed my practice. I now perform over 60 percent of all the surgeries I do robotically, and a straightforward case takes all of 20 minutes. I face the challenging cases with a new mindset. I feel more confident with what I can achieve surgically, knowing I can tackle most cases without making a big incision. What I find most rewarding is when I walk into a patient's room the morning after surgery and she smiles at me and says, "Doc, this is incredible. I'm telling all my friends to have their hysterectomy this way." It's a very good feeling to know that her fears are alleviated, and she can look forward to getting on with her life as quickly as possible. For me, robotic surgery means I spend less time making rounds and more time enjoying pleasant follow-up visits with my patients. The patients are happier, and I am happier! Everybody wins!

Since incorporating robotic surgery into my practice, my thinking about surgery and about my patients as individuals has changed, too. After doing thousands of operations, it's easy to start taking the whole process for granted. Before 2005, in the operating room, my head, my thinking, and my vision were boxed in my patients' bodies, like a portrait photographer with her head inside a blind. Robotic surgery made me step back and see the bigger picture. I had to think about how the machine, my movements, and all the people in the room interacted with my patients on the outside as well as the on the inside. By applying this new tool to more situations, I found myself thinking about how surgery affects each woman individually. I began mentally preparing for these interactions when I saw each patient in the office. I started asking myself, "What can I do to make the experience better for the woman sitting in front of me today? Will my surgery help her feel better? How will what I do affect her job, her family, her relationship with her spouse, and her feelings about her body?"

Finally, gaining expertise and renown with robotic surgery helped me heal from the wounds of misplaced trust. After the breakup of my practice, I had lost faith in people, in medicine, and in myself. By going back to the drawing board and learning something new, I had to humble myself in the operating room during a time when I already felt stripped bare and exposed. I felt ashamed of what had happened, of losing my practice so abruptly. By rebuilding my practice from the ground up, I also rebuilt my own foundation of strength. I learned something that helped more women than ever before in more ways than I had imagined. I loved medicine again.

Most importantly, I learned to love my patients even more for the lessons they teach me every day.

Chapter 2

NOT YOUR MOTHER'S HYSTERECTOMY:

AN INTRODUCTION TO THE MODERN ERA

When I first met Roni Lowery in my office, she had that look I've seen so many times before: that "Please tell me I don't have cancer" look.

"Hi, I'm Dr. Kowalski," I said, my large hand enveloping hers in our handshake. We sat together in my consultation room around a small table. She leaned forward in her chair with her hands clasped tightly, her bright green eyes begging for a shred of good news. With her curly blond hair, infectious smile, and New York accent, she was a woman who usually lights up a room. But that day, she seemed small and frail.

"I haven't been feeling well for a while, but I shrugged it off," she admitted. "I thought the bleeding and pain were probably just my same old ovarian cysts acting up again." But the symptoms got worse. She felt pain under her right breast. She couldn't take a deep breath. Lying on her right side became unbearable.

She made up innocuous explanations in her head: maybe it's a urinary tract infection or a flu bug. Or maybe a pulled muscle.

"Finally, it got so bad that I went to the emergency room. The doctor there told me I had a large cyst on my left ovary, opposite of the side with the pain. He said I should see my gynecologist right away."

At this point, she still didn't think it could be anything serious. But when her gynecologist said he didn't like the way her ovary looked, she began to worry.

"He sent me to the lab to have that blood test for ovarian cancer, the CA-125?" She looked at me for confirmation.

I nodded. This test is ordered when ovarian cancer is suspected.

"Then I had to wait for the results," she said. "I was on pins and needles."

A few days later, an old friend came from Los Angeles for moral support, and the two went straight to the lab to get the results. I glanced at Roni's file as she took a deep breath: her CA-125 level was 190 units/mL, with a normal level being between 0 and 30 units/mL.

"That's when it hit me," Roni said. "Oh, my God, I have cancer! I'm going to need a hysterectomy, just like my mother had. I went out to my car and just bawled."

Roni spoke to her gynecologist on the phone, who referred her to a gynecologic oncologist, a cancer surgeon. With her friend for moral support, she went to see him the next day. But she felt very uncomfortable at the visit.

"He was so cold and matter of fact. My friend thought so, too," she shared as if we were old friends. "But the worst part was that he wouldn't answer my questions. He made me feel stupid for asking them."

"What were your questions?" I asked.

"I wanted to know if I could have the surgery laparoscopically, so I'd have tiny incisions," she explained. "Some of my friends told me that a hysterectomy was possible this way, and I'm afraid of being cut wide open."

"And what did the doctor say?"

Roni made a face. "That he would *try*, but he couldn't promise anything. To be honest, I didn't think he really would try. He just seemed so pessimistic about my chances of avoiding the Big Cut. I've had two cesarean sections, and he said he expected to find scar tissue."

Roni walked out of that visit feeling convinced he was going to open her up no matter what. The thought of putting her life in his hands, under anesthesia and out of control, made her queasy.

Out in her car again, she and her friend decided they needed a second opinion. Roni called another physician who recommended she come see me. Before she walked into my office, she felt positive she had cancer. Why else would they want to cut her wide open? But she also felt a lot of pressure to recover quickly. She needed to drive her daughter, a budding actress, back and forth to auditions in Los Angeles, and was anxious to get back to her life.

Roni's mother Fran, now in her late seventies, had an old-fashioned open hysterectomy 30 years ago. She had painful fibroids and had put off surgery for years. Then she began having severe pelvic pressure. She visited several doctors, hoping one would tell her she didn't need a hysterectomy. She was afraid of "going under" for what seemed like such a big operation. What frightened her most was the risk of complications. She was worried about the wound, about an injury to her internal organs, and about being dependent on her husband until she was better. Would she ever be the same again? A hysterectomy seemed so invasive, and many of her friends had suffered through a difficult recovery. After the operation, Fran spent about a week in the hospital in a great deal of pain. When friends came to visit, she just wanted them to leave so she could be alone and cry. She was told to resume normal activities such as driving, washing dishes, and exercise after eight weeks. But her stitches ripped open. She was afraid and disgusted when she saw all that blood and tissue. The wound took a long time to heal, and even now, years later, she still feels disappointed in the appearance of her scar. Her body felt disfigured. She didn't feel as feminine anymore. Now she was worried when she heard her daughter would need a hysterectomy, too. Would Roni have to go through the same thing? What if Roni had cancer? That would be even worse than what Fran went through.

The other doctor had painted such a scary picture of the surgery that Roni already feared the worst.

"Cancer is only one explanation for your symptoms," I reassured her. I went through the different possibilities with her, explaining that ovarian masses can come from benign tumors, endometriosis, precancers, or cancer. "Until we remove the mass in the operating room, we can only guess at the answer," I told her.

I recommended a robotic hysterectomy and removal of the ovaries and tubes. "I have performed hundreds of these surgeries through several small incisions. The advantages include less pain, a shorter hospital stay, a faster recovery, and a lower risk of complications."

Roni nodded in agreement with the plan.

We would have the mass looked at by the pathologist while she was still under anesthesia and get an answer in just a few minutes. If cancer were identified, then we would have to open her abdomen and check for spread the old-fashioned way. But if the mass was from one of the other non-malignant diseases, then we could save her the Big Cut she feared so much. I explained how we would handle each of the different scenarios in the operating room and how that would affect her recovery. She wanted to know about chemotherapy and cancer survival, but I suggested we wait until after the surgery.

"What if we never need to have that conversation?" I asked.

Her eyes brightened with surprise and new hope. "You mean there's really a chance it might not be cancer?"

"Yes, there is a chance," I said, "but we will be ready to handle whatever we find."

For the first time since she entered my office, Roni's face relaxed. She smiled a little. "Thank you for listening to me," she said.

She was anxious to have the surgery right away, so we scheduled her for the following week. When I shook her hand goodbye and looked into her eyes, her relief and confidence in me shone back. This time, she walked out of the doctor's office feeling hopeful and safe. As a surgeon, there is no better reward than inspiring confidence in my patients. I was so gratified that Roni knew in her heart I would make the right decisions for her, no matter what we found in the operating room.

Surgery for ovarian masses reminds me of that line from Forrest Gump when his mother says, "Life is like a box of chocolates. You never know what you're gonna get." The same is true in the operating room. The moment of truth comes when we first put the camera in the belly and everyone in the room sees what's inside. In Roni's case, the first view looked ugly. Her organs looked glued together and distorted. We saw bands of scar tissue from her previous cesarean sections. Her ovaries were no longer recognizable, replaced by tumors that appeared swollen and ominous. Despite this, we were safely able to remove everything using the small incisions. We placed the tumors in a special bag, brought them out through the vagina, and sent them off to the lab. I scrubbed out and walked down the hall to the pathology suite, where the pathologist and I examined the tumors together. Looking through the microscope is a window into a tumor's personality, so I like to get that picture in my head to understand each case more thoroughly. In Roni's case, the picture was initially not so clear. We saw definite signs of abnormal cells, but no obvious cancer. We looked at some more sections, and still no cancer. The answer came into focus: it was precancer. She didn't need the Big Cut. By removing her tumors, Roni was cured. I couldn't wait to tell her.

Later that afternoon, I visited her in her hospital bed.

"Roni, everything's going to be okay. No cancer," I said, smiling.

At first, she looked up at me unsurely. Then the relief and joy crossed her face, replacing all the worry as her recovery officially began.

Getting back to her normal life was a breeze. "Night and day," she said, compared to her C-sections. She only took her narcotic pain pills for a few days and was walking right away. By her six-week checkup, the cancer scare seemed a million miles away. Her mother, Fran, was amazed at the difference compared to her experience years ago. Now Roni wants other women to know what she went through, so they can learn from her experiences. Roni's story is familiar to many women because hysterectomy is so common. That is the reason I am writing this book.

. . .

Hysterectomy is the second most common operation performed on women in the United States, eclipsed only by the cesarean section. Faced with the prospect of surgery, many women are unaware of the medical choices available today. To arrive at the best decision, you and your doctor must sort through these choices together. Although many excellent books are available to help guide you, none do so in this modern era of medical technology—the era of robotics. There are so many options out there; how do you choose? Most women just follow their doctor's advice, without understanding the reasoning behind the recommendation.

For women of any age, hysterectomy is a last resort when a healthy life is at stake. Fortunately, the uterus makes no hormones and does not contribute to any vital bodily function required for survival. The only physiological purpose of the uterus is to carry a pregnancy. Therefore, if a medical condition requires hysterectomy for treatment, a woman can continue leading a healthy life without her uterus. Of course, she cannot carry a pregnancy afterward, but, fortunately, most conditions that require a hysterectomy occur later in life, after the opportunity for childbearing has already passed. Nobody *wants* to have a hysterectomy unless it's absolutely necessary, but sometimes it is. Despite what many women think, doctors are not hungry to take organs out just for the money or some sense of power or ego. The vast majority of doctors want to help people, and they know from their training and experience that, for some problems, taking out the uterus will help best.

The medical term "hysterectomy" refers to the surgical removal of the uterus with its attached cervix. In the plainest terms, that is all the word means and no more. However, what may be more important is what it *doesn't* mean. To explain, it does not mean removing the ovaries and/or tubes. That is a separate operation called a bilateral salpingo-oophorectomy, which is frequently performed at the same time as a hysterectomy. It also does not include a bladder lift or a vaginal repair. It does, however, include removal of the cervix.

I spend a great deal of time in my practice offering consultations about hysterectomy. Most women come to me already knowing they need a hysterectomy. A big part of my job during these initial consultations is to come up with a surgical game plan. I ask questions, review test results, perform a physical exam, and then I think through the options. When I sit down with the patient, I want to get a sense of how the surgery will affect the woman sitting in front of me. What can I do to help her problem? How can I make this process as easy on her as possible? What surgical option is the best choice for her? I call this mental process "Surgeon's Logic," because it is how surgeons are trained to think. Going through these decision points daily in my practice, I have tried to find ways to convey my Surgeon's Logic to patients. Now, with this book, I hope to convey this reasoning to you.

Many women are afraid to have a hysterectomy, even when they know it's necessary. They remember what their mothers went through. They wonder if they will feel the same afterward. Fears about sexuality are common. "Will I still feel like a woman?" is a frequent question. If you need a hysterectomy, presumably there is a problem causing symptoms or discomfort. Abnormal bleeding and pain are not very conducive to a healthy sex life. Research shows that women generally report an *improvement* in their sex life after hysterectomy, because whatever caused them to seek medical attention in the first place is now gone. With the bleeding stopped, you can feel like yourself again.

Every woman is a unique individual, so what is best for one could be dangerous for another. When I meet with a patient in the office, the better informed she is, the better job I can do discussing the different options. Together, we can develop a treatment plan that fits the individual. That way, when the day of surgery arrives, she can go into the operating room feeling confident that I will perform the best surgery for her. I believe this is a superior way to provide health care compared to the more patronizing approach from the past. I can't tell you how many patients I see who had a hysterectomy years ago, and they don't know why or how it was done. Most aren't sure what parts were removed.

"Do you know why you had a hysterectomy?" I ask.

"My doctor just said I needed it," is the answer.

"Do you know how it was done?" I also want to know.

"They said it was a partial," I hear.

At this point, *I* become confused, because partial hysterectomy is a layperson's term, not a medical term. When a woman tells me this, I really don't know what she had done.

"Do you have any records from that surgery?" I ask hopefully.

She admits, "Nobody gave me any records. What kind of records?"

We resign ourselves to being left in the dark. Neither my patient nor I will ever know what was done to her body. In this day and age, we can do better.

This is a revolutionary time for women's health. Life expectancy for women is at its highest ever, over 80 years. Many women will live well into their nineties. What about the quality of those years? What can we do to make those years satisfying and fulfilling? We are all busier than ever before, and we have higher expectations of ourselves and our lives. No longer are the twenty-somethings the only entrants in a local triathlon. No longer are men the only top executives in business. Life does not stop and wait for us to catch up.

So what do you do if you find yourself in a situation like Roni Lowery's? You are in pain, you're scared, and you just want to feel better. You go to the doctor and hope for the best. You want to find a good doctor, one who can explain things to you, who is a competent surgeon, and who will guide you through your recovery. How daunting it must be to come to the doctor's office and have no idea what's wrong with you or how to fix it.

Surgeons see these things every day. Sometimes we forget what it's like to be the patient, feeling vulnerable and scared. For you, the patient, to feel empowered, you need some knowledge and insight into the process. You need to know enough about your condition for an individualized solution to make sense. You need some tips to help you choose the right doctor, and you need an understanding of your surgical choices. Let's sit down together and dive in.

Chapter 3

ANATOMY 101

How well do you know your anatomy? If you're like many of my patients, you may have learned it in a high school health class and long since shelved that knowledge. Other patients of mine *never* learned it. The truth is that, yes, anatomy can be complex. But understanding it will help you understand how your body works as we delve into specific surgical treatments, and its terminology will give you the language to feel empowered in your appointments with your doctor.

Like an opera in a foreign language, if you don't know the background of the story, you can't follow the plot and won't get much out of the performance. Let's create the scene for a hysterectomy so you can follow along. The backdrop is the female pelvis, where the organs reside. The terminology is the language, and the surgical principles are the scaffolding upon which the story unfolds. So, while this chapter is detailed, stick with me for the basic information you need to know. For more detailed definitions, see the glossary of terms at the end of this book.

First, let's take a look at figures 1 and 2 of the reproductive organs that we commonly refer to in gynecologic surgery. The uterus takes center stage in the picture—normally a lemon-sized organ, it sits between the bladder in front and the colon behind. The ovaries are small, whitish organs, about the size of a prune. Fallopian tubes resemble the size and shape of green beans. The ovaries and fallopian tubes come off each side of the uterus, but they also attach to their own blood vessels from the sides of the pelvis. Also, notice how the uterus and cervix form one continuous organ. In fact, the term *cervix* is Latin for neck and simply refers to the neck or narrow part of the uterus.

Let's review the important structures in figures 1 and 2:

- **Fallopian tubes:** tubes that pass the eggs released from the ovaries during ovulation into the uterine cavity.
- **Ovaries:** small, whitish-colored organs containing all the eggs a woman has from birth. They also produce most of a woman's sex hormones.

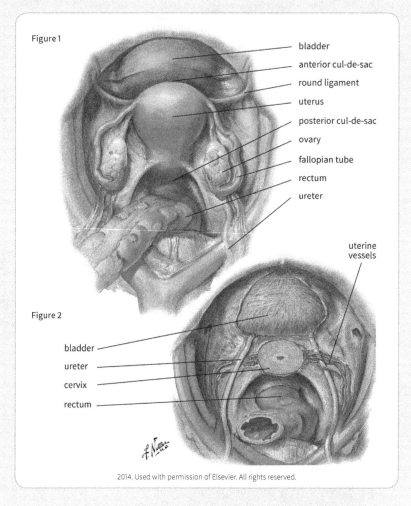

Figure 1

- bladder
- anterior cul-de-sac
- round ligament
- uterus
- posterior cul-de-sac
- ovary
- fallopian tube
- rectum
- ureter

uterine vessels

Figure 2

- bladder
- ureter
- cervix
- rectum

Figure 1 represents a view of the pelvic organs from the perspective of a camera placed in the belly button looking down into the pelvis. The bladder is front and center. The reproductive organs sit in the middle. The colon and rectum fill the backside. Notice how the ureters run along the sides of the uterus and into the bladder just next to the cervix. It's also important to see that the blood supply to all the pelvic organs comes from each side toward the center. The major arteries are red and the veins blue.

Figure 2 is an artist's rendering of how some of the critical structures in the pelvis relate to each other. To do this, the smooth peritoneal lining covering all the structures has been stripped away, the colon has been divided at the top of the pelvis, and the top of the uterus has been separated from the cervix. The purpose of this view is to demonstrate the relationship of the uterine blood supply to the ureters and bladder. This perspective is not meant to suggest that this is how we see things during surgery, but it will help you understand the anatomic relationships of some of the important structures we will be discussing throughout the course of this book.

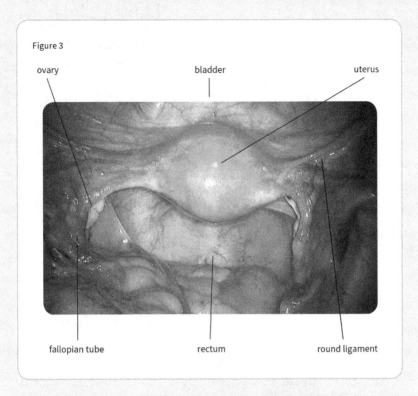

Figure 3

ovary   bladder   uterus

fallopian tube   rectum   round ligament

Figure 3 shows a photograph of normal female pelvic anatomy, again from the perspective of a camera inserted in the belly button. This is the view the surgeon sees during pelvic laparoscopy. Notice how all the organs appear smooth and proportional. Also notice that the blood vessels and ureters are not visible, because they are covered in the normal peritoneal lining. During surgery, the blood vessels and other critical structures must be dissected free from the tissue surrounding them to safely perform the operation.

- **Uterus:** the muscular organ in the middle of the pelvis where pregnancies develop. Also known as the "womb." When we say uterus, we are usually referring to both the uterus and cervix as one organ.
- **Cervix:** the narrow part at the bottom of the uterus. This is the area that dilates during childbirth to allow the baby to pass through the birth canal.
- **Vagina:** this muscular tube forms the birth canal.
- **Anterior cul-de-sac:** the space between the bladder and uterus.
- **Posterior cul-de-sac:** the space between the uterus and rectum.

Now compare the drawings in figures 1 and 2 to the photograph of a normal woman's pelvis in figure 3. This is exactly what I see when I look inside a woman's body at the start of a pelvic operation. If there is something abnormal with the organs, like fibroids or a mass, the picture will look much different. Notice how the organs are pink and smooth. The yellow areas are fat, which is normally stored around the colon and intestines. When I perform a hysterectomy, my goal is to remove the uterus but leave surrounding organs, like the bladder and rectum, unharmed.

Don't worry: you will not be tested on where your round ligaments or ureter or colon are. Having an awareness of their location, and more importantly, having a resource to know more about them and how they function, is most essential. These figures are just to get you started.

In the back of the book, you'll find a more extensive glossary of terms. Feel free to refer to this more expanded list as we continue through our journey. You can also visit my website, *http://www.not yourmothershysterectomy.com*, for pictures of abnormal organs to compare to the normal pictures you see here.

Chapter 4

"WHAT BRINGS YOU IN TO SEE ME TODAY?"
YOUR SYMPTOMS TELL THE STORY

When something goes wrong with your body, it's often a gradual process. You might notice that a little something doesn't seem right one day, but by the next day it's gone. Then, if it comes back or gets worse, you may start to wonder if it's serious. You may go to the doctor or even your local emergency room. Tests ensue, and before you know it, a whole story unfolds. That story, your story, matters to your doctor. The narrative of your symptoms tells us a lot about you and your health.

In this chapter, we will discuss the most common symptoms that may require hysterectomy for treatment. In the next chapter, we will delve into the causes of those symptoms—the medical conditions that produce them. To distinguish, symptoms are the feelings or changes you experience in your body, whereas conditions or diagnoses define the *cause* of those symptoms. For example, remember Roni Lowery from chapter 2? She was feeling pain on her right side and experiencing abnormal bleeding. Those were her symptoms. When I saw her in my office, my working diagnosis was a pelvic mass. After I removed the mass and it was processed in the pathology laboratory, the final diagnosis (cause) was a precancerous tumor of her ovaries. The condition that caused of all her symptoms was the tumor.

For simplicity at this point in the book, I will refer to all types of hysterectomy together as just "hysterectomy." Some of the information in this chapter may not relate to your specific concerns. I encourage you to browse through the different areas for what seems relevant, but don't feel obligated to read everything presented here. If you relate to any of these symptoms, use that section to learn more about what you are feeling. Please remember, though, that an individualized assessment of *your* symptoms is beyond the scope of a book and that only your doctor can diagnose your specific condition after a full evaluation.

Now, what are the common symptoms women experience when something is wrong with their reproductive organs? These are the things you, the patient, tell me when I ask my standard go-to question: "So what brings you in to see me today?" The four most common answers are abnormal bleeding, pelvic pain, pelvic masses, and pelvic prolapse.

Very often, these symptoms overlap. For example, abnormal bleeding commonly causes a cramping type of pain. A mass can be associated with abnormal bleeding and pain. Chronic inflammation from prolapse (when the pelvic organs start to fall out through the vagina) can sometimes lead to abnormal bleeding. Pressure from a large mass can cause prolapse. Let's break down each symptom individually to better explain.

ABNORMAL BLEEDING

Abnormal bleeding is the most common gynecologic symptom treated by hysterectomy. Abnormal periods in premenopausal women can be from many causes but are quite different from bleeding after menopause. *Any* bleeding after menopause is considered abnormal and should be immediately evaluated by your doctor. Persistent bleeding after intercourse is also abnormal and should be evaluated.

"Dr. Kowalski, I am bleeding fifteen days out of every month and passing huge clots," Connie, a 45-year-old cashier, told me when we sat down to talk. A short, dark-haired Hispanic woman, Connie looked pale and exhausted to me, and it came as no surprise: normal periods in a premenopausal woman should come every 22–36 days and should last no longer than seven days. How much bleeding constitutes abnormal bleeding is hard to quantify. Most women have an idea from their own experience when their bleeding is too much, and Connie had long since reached that point.

"I have had difficult periods all my life, but the last year has been unbearable." Her voice cracked. "Sometimes I go through 10 pads a day. I can't make it through my shift at work, I don't have any energy for exercise, and it hurts to have sex with my husband."

"Okay, Connie," I told her. "Let's figure out what's going on here."

Connie's description of her symptoms led me to suspect she had uterine fibroids, and my suspicion was confirmed when I examined her. At the time of surgery, her uterus was enlarged to the size of a grapefruit. Once she had her hysterectomy, she gave all her tampons and pads away.

When I asked Geneva, a 62-year-old retired schoolteacher, my go-to opening question, she admitted to bleeding for the last six months.

"First it started as a little brown staining in my underwear. Now I see red blood on some days and nothing other days," she explained.

Geneva had uterine cancer, the most serious cause of postmenopausal bleeding. At just over five feet tall and over 250 pounds, she was nervous about her risks of having a big cancer operation. She didn't have any other symptoms, such as pain or trouble going to the bathroom, so I was hopeful her cancer had not spread beyond her uterus.

"You are an excellent candidate for minimally invasive surgery," I told her. She was so relieved to know that she didn't need a big incision, her eyes welled up and she gave me a big hug.

The evaluation for abnormal bleeding typically includes a complete history and physical examination, Pap smear, and pelvic ultrasound. During the physical exam, your doctor will want to examine the vulva, vagina, and cervix to look for any obvious source of the bleeding. When your doctor feels the cervix, uterus, and ovaries, she is checking for any enlargement or mass. Depending on her suspicion for precancer or cancer, she may also recommend an office endometrial biopsy or a dilation and curettage (D and C), which is done in the operating room.

A pelvic ultrasound is usually the best imaging study to view the female reproductive organs. These can be done in two ways: an abdominal version similar to scanning a pregnant woman's belly, and a transvaginal exam using a slender probe inserted in the vagina. A transvaginal study, although less comfortable than a standard abdominal ultrasound, is more accurate in evaluating the female organs. If the abdominal ultrasound doesn't show anything to explain the bleeding, a transvaginal study needs to be done anyway. And if the abdominal ultrasound shows a fibroid, mass, or other abnormality, a transvaginal ultrasound will show the same findings with more accuracy. So my advice is: request the transvaginal study from the start.

Abnormal bleeding does not always come from the uterus. A problem with the cervix or in the vagina can also cause bleeding. Bleeding after intercourse is sometimes caused by a cervical mass. A problem on the vulva, such as vulvar cancer or vulvar ulceration, can also cause bleeding. Finally, bleeding from the bladder, rectum, or anus can be mistaken for uterine bleeding. The important point here is that the bleeding can't be ignored; it must be accounted for. If a basic workup does not reveal the cause, you and your doctor must investigate other possible sources until a diagnosis is reached.

PELVIC PAIN

Pelvic pain is an enormously complex problem affecting many women. Pain can be sharp, dull, or crampy, and it can be cyclical, intermittent, or constant. Pain is obviously a very personal state—what some women describe as pain, others would call pressure or discomfort.

The type of pain you feel might vary based on your condition. Pain with your menstrual period is most likely related to a gynecologic condition, but chronic pelvic pain can be related to non-gynecologic problems as well. Common gynecologic conditions such as uterine fibroids or endometriosis often cause an uncomfortable feeling of fullness and pressure in addition to menstrual pain. Meanwhile, most women describe the sensation of pelvic prolapse as a feeling of pressure more than pain, and while precancerous conditions do not cause pain, any type of cancer can. We will discuss all these conditions in more detail in upcoming sections.

Jane, a 36-year-old social worker, explained her pain like this: "It's like there's a tight banjo string inside my stomach. I feel it vibrate and pull. When my period comes, it gets unbearable. I have to take off work and just lie in bed until it's over."

Jane's pain came from endometriosis. A slight, fit-appearing woman, she felt disfigured by all the scars on her abdomen. She had previously undergone several laparoscopic surgeries to remove deposits of endometriosis in her pelvis. She also tried controlling the symptoms with birth control pills and an IUD. She had gone through so much already, trying to avoid a hysterectomy. But her symptoms kept getting worse, and she had to listen to what her body was telling her. Ultimately, when all other treatments failed, hysterectomy was her last resort.

The non-gynecologic causes of pelvic pain are numerous, including conditions affecting the urinary, digestive, lymphatic, vascular, musculoskeletal, or neurologic systems. A discussion of these areas is beyond the scope of this book, but other symptoms that accompany the pain will often suggest one cause over another. For example, pelvic pain that occurs with rectal bleeding is more likely to be from colorectal disease than a gynecologic problem. Pain associated with blood in the urine could be a kidney stone or from bladder cancer.

Pain is generally a sign of a problem and should be investigated. Your doctor will probably want to perform a complete history and physical examination, laboratory testing such as blood work or urinalysis, and some type of imaging study. Either a pelvic ultrasound, computed tomography (CT) scan, or magnetic resonance imaging (MRI) scan may be the best test, depending on the other characteristics of your condition.

PELVIC MASSES

Pelvic masses commonly lead to a visit with a surgeon. Many women who feel a lump or mass in their pelvic area tell me they happened to find it while lying in bed. Others notice their stomach getting bigger despite trying to lose weight. Some describe a heavy feeling, as though they're carrying something extra around inside of them. These symptoms can be associated with constipation and/or a feeling of urinary urgency or frequency. All of these feelings can be caused by a pelvic mass.

Nancy, a middle-aged real estate agent, said, "I just thought I was getting fat. I couldn't understand why my stomach kept getting bigger, even though I was working out all the time. Then I couldn't catch my breath when I bent over to pick something up." She added, "It feels like something is sitting on my bladder all the time. I have to pee about every two hours."

Nancy's mass was from a benign ovarian tumor the size of a cantaloupe.

In many cases, a healthcare provider finds a mass during a routine physical exam when the patient doesn't realize she has one. She may have vague symptoms or no symptoms at all without noticing an actual lump. Regardless of the symptoms, any pelvic mass requires further evaluation.

The word "mass" sounds frightening, but in reality, it is a very general term and simply means there is a lump. The phrase "pelvic mass" can be used to describe a growth such as a cyst, tumor, or fibroid. The word *cyst* refers to a fluid-filled mass. *Tumors* are growths that can be benign, premalignant, or malignant. But a pelvic mass could also come from a foreign body, an overfilled bladder, retained stool, or even a developing pregnancy. The term *pelvic mass*, therefore, simply refers to the presence of a lump in the pelvis. A bit like a detective, part of a doctor's job is to find the culprit.

The sleuthing process for determining the cause of any symptom is called a "workup." The workup of a pelvic mass includes a thorough history and physical examination, Pap smear, blood work, and then usually a CT scan of the abdomen and pelvis. A CT scan is preferable to an ultrasound in this case because it provides a view of all the abdominal and pelvic organs. Without yet knowing the source of the mass, the doctor is in detective mode, exploring possible suspects. In addition, one mass might signify the presence of other masses. A CT scan can identify other associated masses more thoroughly than an ultrasound.

One of the first things I think about when seeing a woman with a mass is whether she is pre- or postmenopausal. When a menstruating woman ovulates each month, one of her ovaries produces a small cyst around the egg called a follicular cyst. However, a follicular cyst is not pathologic (abnormal) and is a *normal* part of reproductive function. Because postmenopausal women no longer ovulate, any mass is considered pathologic (abnormal). But, as you will see, not all masses need to be surgically removed.

With the results of your imaging study in hand, your doctor must then interpret them in light of your individual case. For example, let's say that the CT scan shows a growth in the reproductive organs. Certain characteristics of a mass may *suggest* one diagnosis over another. No imaging study on its own can make a diagnosis. A scan shows characteristics of a mass, but only a laboratory analysis by a pathologist can give us the true diagnosis. Just like a crime scene investigation, a team of doctors works together to find the culprit. Pathologic masses usually appear complex on imaging studies, with fluid-filled and solid areas. Some masses are completely solid. A mass may have an irregular shape or appear attached to other structures. These characteristics can be seen on the scan and will significantly influence the recommendations for treatment. For example, a solitary mass in a young woman may be removed through a few small incisions without hysterectomy, while a suspicious mass in an older woman may require more extensive surgery. For this reason, women with masses suspicious for cancer should be referred to a gynecologic oncologist, a cancer specialist like me.

Some blood tests can be helpful in assessing the level of suspicion for cancer. The CA-125 level is one such test. CA-125 is the name for a protein made by the cells lining your peritoneal cavity (the space containing your abdominal and pelvic organs). CA-125 can be measured in the blood, where a small amount, usually 0–30 units/mL, is normally present. Some cancers produce large amounts of this protein, but other conditions can increase the level as well. Roni Lowery's CA-125 was elevated at 190 units/mL, raising suspicion of cancer. But ultimately, she did not have cancer. The inflammation from her precancerous tumors caused her abdominal cavity to produce an abnormal amount of this protein.

Other non-cancerous conditions can cause the body to produce an excess amount of CA-125. This is common with cirrhosis of the liver, appendicitis, endometriosis, and even fibroids. It's best to think of the CA-125 as a piece of information in the overall puzzle, but it should not be given more weight than it's worth. The CA-125 is not always elevated in cases of cancer and sometimes is elevated from conditions other than cancer. Therefore, it is not a critical element of the decision-making process but can be a useful piece of information in the overall assessment of a patient's case. An elevated CA-125 in a woman with ovarian cancer can be used as a marker to follow her response to treatment. That's why we want to check it before surgery to know our starting point.

The size of a pelvic mass is also important. Larger masses are more likely to require surgical removal. In general, a simple fluid-filled cyst less than five centimeters (almost two inches) in a postmenopausal woman is very *unlikely* to be cancer and often will just be observed. One of the first questions I ask a woman in this circumstance is, "Are you having pain from this? Does the mass bother you?" If not, surgery is often best avoided.

For example, I see Betty every six months or so. She is a 75-year-old white-haired woman who's a little hard of hearing and typically comes to the appointment with her daughter. Betty was referred to me with a 4.8 cm simple fluid-filled cyst. She would have never known it was there if it weren't for an MRI she had after a car accident. These small cysts are not typically suspicious for cancer. But if the cyst starts to cause her pain or gets larger over time, then it's going to need to come out. Her lack of symptoms from the cyst is reassuring, and hers hasn't grown over the last year and a half. Each time I see her and tell her she is still okay, she claps her hands together and says, "No surgery? No problem!"

The larger the mass, the more likely surgery is necessary. Anything larger than about eight centimeters (almost four inches) in a premenopausal woman and anything larger than five centimeters (between two and three inches) in a postmenopausal woman must be removed to rule out cancer. In addition, larger masses are more likely to rupture, twist, or cause pain by pressing against other organs. Surgical removal is usually the best treatment to relieve these symptoms.

Depending on the location of the mass, a biopsy prior to definitive surgical removal may not be advisable. For example, if the mass involves one or both ovaries, a biopsy is not recommended for several reasons. The ovaries share the same space in our abdominal cavity as our intestines and other internal organs. Sticking a needle through the abdominal wall and into the ovary risks injuring the bowels. But more importantly, puncturing the ovary to get a biopsy can spill the contents of whatever is contained inside the mass. In the case of many benign or malignant tumors, infections, or endometriosis, this should be avoided. In addition, a biopsy does not change the course of action to treat the mass. Regardless of the result of the biopsy, surgery is still required to remove it. Finally, masses can be composed of different types of tissue in different areas. A biopsy of one part of a mass may show a benign tumor when right next to that spot may be another area containing cancer. The only way to definitively know the nature of a mass is to remove it entirely and have a pathologist analyze it microscopically. Therefore, in most cases, surgery is the recommended treatment to both diagnose and remove a pelvic mass.

PELVIC PROLAPSE

Pelvic prolapse is another symptom many women experience. They may not call it by that name, but they often use the phrase, "I feel something falling out of my vagina" to describe prolapse. Many women with prolapse also feel a constant pressure in the vagina that gets worse throughout the day.

Prolapse results from a progressive weakening of the pelvic tissues. The pelvic organs don't hold themselves in place. Instead, the strong muscles and ligaments of the pelvic floor provide support for the internal organs. Over time, a damaged pelvic floor, usually from the trauma of childbirth, becomes weak until the organs of the pelvis succumb to the force of gravity. In severe cases, some women can feel their uterus extending beyond the vaginal opening and hanging between their legs. Many women with prolapse notice problems with urination, not realizing that pelvic floor weakness is the root cause.

The term *prolapse* refers to both the symptoms and the condition. Any number of organs can prolapse out the vaginal opening, including the bladder, the intestines, the rectum, and even the vagina itself. The symptoms usually develop slowly over several years and, although not inherently dangerous, can be debilitating. The type of prolapse depends on which other organs are involved. The symptoms of prolapse are commonly associated with urinary incontinence, constipation, and vaginal inflammation. Most cases involve more than one organ, so a full evaluation is necessary to treat the entire problem.

This evaluation includes, at the start, a complete physical examination. Prolapse is easily seen by your doctor with a pelvic examination. Very often, simply bearing down during the exam will cause the weakened tissues to bulge outward. Additional testing, such as pelvic ultrasound, urodynamics, defecography, dynamic MRI scan, or 3-D pelvic floor ultrasound may provide valuable insight into different aspects of the problem. Urinary symptoms commonly accompany prolapse, and urodynamics are an important component of the evaluation. The term *urodynamics* describes a series of tests to measure how the bladder fills and empties. These tests can help your doctor determine the exact nature of your problem and then recommend the best treatment.

We have discussed the four most common gynecologic symptoms associated with the need for hysterectomy, but other symptoms such as abnormal vaginal discharge, a change in bowel habits, bloating, or change in urinary habits can also suggest a problem. The symptoms you feel are the reason you visit your doctor to begin with, but they also point her in the right direction to find the cause. Take the time to listen to your body and describe your symptoms to her in as much detail as possible. Discussing your symptoms probably feels vulnerable, but it allows your doctor to start formulating a treatment plan. By listening to you and educating you, she should help alleviate your worries. To continue arming you with the knowledge you need to approach your care with confidence, the next chapter will address the causes for your symptoms and explain why and when hysterectomy may be the best option.

Chapter 5

SO YOU THINK YOU NEED A HYSTERECTOMY:
THE WHY BEHIND YOUR OPERATION

In the last chapter, we explored the variety of symptoms that might bring you in to see your doctor. Conditions causing disease in the reproductive organs create these symptoms. Doctors can sometimes treat these conditions with medications or other non-invasive interventions, but for many diseases, hysterectomy offers the best long-term solution. For benign conditions like uterine fibroids or endometriosis, hysterectomy is usually a last resort. But for life-threatening diseases like cancer, surgery is often the only option for cure.

When something feels wrong with your body, you go to your doctor in search of answers. How does your doctor arrive at those answers? As we discussed in the previous chapter, the story of your symptoms points us in the right direction. A physical examination adds more pieces to the puzzle. Laboratory tests and imaging studies help bring greater clarity to the picture. Ultimately, our goal is to identify the *cause* of your symptoms, the condition that started the whole problem to begin with. Then we can recommend appropriate treatment to heal that condition. In other words, the "why" behind your hysterectomy starts here.

With this chapter, I will briefly discuss some alternatives to hysterectomy, but a more thorough discussion is beyond my intended purpose. There are good sources you can refer to for more information about these alternatives. I certainly am not suggesting that every woman with the conditions we will talk about needs a hysterectomy. My intention is to help you understand your own situation better *if* you need a hysterectomy, presuming you have already explored alternative treatments.

This chapter will be most helpful to you if your doctor has already established your diagnosis and you have questions about your condition and your treatment options. I have broken down these conditions into benign and malignant categories to simplify their explanation.

BENIGN INDICATIONS FOR HYSTERECTOMY

The term *benign* means "not cancer," and, in my line of work as an oncologist, it's my favorite word. As with Roni Lowery, many women go into surgery not knowing if they have cancer or not. After the operation, when we have that first conversation about the findings, there's a lot of relief and often tears of joy when I can use the word *benign*.

FIBROIDS

By far, the most common condition treated by hysterectomy is fibroids. Uterine fibroids are benign tumors of the uterine muscle that can cause abnormal bleeding, pain, and/or infertility. Because they come from the uterine wall, as they grow and enlarge, the uterus becomes enlarged along with them. Each individual fibroid is a tumor, and often multiple fibroids exist at the same time. Each tumor adds to the size of the uterus, causing enlargement of the uterus as a whole. Some fibroids are very small, the size of a pea. Others are as large as basketballs. In some cases, they can essentially take over the uterus, replacing the normal uterine muscle with multiple fibroid tumors. Because uterine fibroids do not respond predictably to a woman's natural hormonal cycles and because they induce the formation of a rich network of blood vessels, they can cause abnormal and heavy vaginal bleeding.

A fibroid uterus may grow slowly over many years and can lead to debilitating problems. When you are bleeding all the time, it can be hard to work, exercise, or take care of your household. It can also take a toll on your relationships. Connie, the cashier in chapter 4 who was bleeding so frequently, explained to me, "It's hard to feel romantic when you don't even feel clean." Often a partner doesn't understand those feelings, and relationships can suffer. Pain and cramping cause many women to miss work, putting their jobs at stake. Heavy, prolonged bleeding can even be life threatening. Abnormal periods over months or years can lead to anemia, sometimes requiring blood transfusions. I have seen women come to the hospital with blood counts so low from bleeding fibroids that I wonder how they are still alive.

Fibroids cause pain by pressing against other nearby organs. An enlarged fibroid uterus can push against your bladder, making you feel as though you have to pee all the time. It can sit like a heavy weight on your rectum or back, leading to constipation and/or back pain. Fibroids can also make intercourse painful, especially with deep penetration. Larger fibroids take up space in your abdomen, causing bloating, difficulty bending over, or fatigue. Think of it like carrying around an extra weight all day long.

Some fibroids can push against the uterine cavity, affecting fertility. In some cases, they may interfere with getting pregnant by disrupting implantation of an embryo, but more commonly, they lead to pregnancy loss. As the fetus grows, pressure from the fibroid(s) in the uterine wall can push against it, leading to miscarriage.

Many treatments other than hysterectomy exist for fibroids, but ultimately, the fibroids usually recur. This happens because the tumors can grow in any part of the uterine muscle. Until all those muscle fibers are removed, the tumors tend to keep coming back. If you had a skin tumor on your foot, for example, and your doctor just removed part of it, you would expect the remainder to grow back eventually. The same is true for fibroids. In cases where we want to preserve fertility so a woman can have a family, we look for strategies to treat the fibroids for as long as possible without hysterectomy. Some of these strategies include medication, uterine artery embolization, radio-frequency ablation, endometrial ablation, and myomectomy. (These terms are defined in the glossary at the end of this book.)

Most fibroid tumors are responsive to hormones in both positive and negative ways. Estrogen can cause the fibroids to grow. Medications such as leuprolide acetate (Lupron) can shrink the fibroids by suppressing the body's production of estrogen. However, suppressing estrogen essentially puts the body into menopause, with all its associated unpleasant side effects. Treatment with Lupron is only a temporary fix, because a woman cannot take this medication for longer than about six months. This is because a prolonged "medical menopause" in a young woman can lead to severe osteoporosis, not to mention other unpleasant symptoms such as vaginal dryness and hot flashes. Therefore, Lupron is primarily a bridging agent prior to planned surgery rather than a long-term solution. Shrinking larger fibroids with Lupron prior to surgery increases the chance for a less invasive operation with less blood loss but may take months to achieve the desired effect.

A newer option for medical therapy to treat fibroids uses drugs that selectively suppress progesterone receptors in the uterine tissue. Progesterone receptors are the structures on the surface of the uterine cells that recognize the presence of the hormone progesterone and transmit its signal to the rest of the cell. One of these new drugs, ulipristal acetate, has been studied in Europe and shown to decrease bleeding from fibroids with very few of the typical menopausal symptoms of Lupron.

For those young women who cannot tolerate the side effects of Lupron, cannot wait for Lupron to work due to severe symptoms, or have been unresponsive to hormonal treatment in general, myomectomy is sometimes recommended. Myomectomy is the removal of just the fibroid tumor or tumors while leaving the rest of the uterus intact. This procedure is reserved for women who are trying to get pregnant but cannot because of their fibroids.

Myomectomy is not recommended in older women or women who are past childbearing age for several reasons. First, fibroids tend to come back, so myomectomy is only a temporary fix. Second, myomectomy is a more technically difficult and sometimes riskier operation than a hysterectomy. There is typically more bleeding, a longer operative time, and more postoperative pain with myomectomy compared to hysterectomy. Many older women don't understand these issues and come to me requesting a myomectomy to treat fibroids. When I discuss these concerns with them, many patients say they didn't know the fibroids would come back. Again, this stems from the fact that fibroids are, in fact, tumors. The bottom line is this: if having children is *not* in your future, then you are better off with a hysterectomy than a myomectomy.

I don't make this statement lightly. I know it sounds very "surgeon-like," maybe even a bit callous, to recommend taking parts of the body out. But over the years, I have taken care of women who had a myomectomy and were disheartened to learn they would later need another operation because the fibroids usually come back. Although benign tumors are not like cancers that can spread, by their nature, they tend to recur if not completely removed. In addition, myomectomies typically heal with a fair amount of scar tissue, making a future operation potentially riskier. Therefore, if you make the choice for a myomectomy, make sure it is for the right reasons and with a good understanding of the implications of your choice.

A condition similar to fibroids, adenomyosis occurs when there is an overgrowth of the uterine muscle *and* uterine lining. Just like fibroids, adenomyosis can cause abnormal bleeding, uterine enlargement, and pain. In contrast to fibroids, adenomyosis tends to cause the uterus to enlarge symmetrically. Fibroids often grow as lumps and bumps coming off the uterus in odd shapes and angles. Fibroids are easily distinguished from the rest of the uterus on ultrasound, MRI, or CT scan, whereas adenomyosis can appear as a general enlargement of the uterine tissue. Many women have never heard of the term adenomyosis, because it's difficult to identify on an ultrasound and therefore not a word women commonly hear. Ultimately, this condition is best diagnosed once the uterus has been removed and examined under the microscope.

Very often, when a woman has the symptoms of fibroids, such as abnormal bleeding and painful periods, but the ultrasound appears normal, the explanation is adenomyosis. Because of the elusive nature of an adenomyosis diagnosis, many women come to my office for consultation frustrated because they have been told there is nothing wrong with them. They know they have abnormal bleeding and pain, but nothing specific shows up on their ultrasound. Sometimes they are made to feel like it's all in their heads. In these cases, adenomyosis is often the culprit. What a relief for them when we review the pathology report and they realize there was a real explanation for what they were feeling.

ENDOMETRIOSIS

Another common benign reason for hysterectomy is endometriosis. Normally, endometrial tissue lines the inside of the uterine cavity. This is the tissue a woman sheds every month with her menstrual cycle. When this tissue is found anywhere outside of its normal location, we call it endometriosis. This condition affects young, menstruating women.

Although the cause of endometriosis is not completely understood, it is likely related to a woman's response to her own menstrual tissue. Every month when you menstruate, not all of the blood comes out through the vagina. Some of the blood backs up through the fallopian tubes and into the pelvis. On many occasions, I have performed laparoscopy on women during their period. As soon as I place the camera inside the abdomen, I can see menstrual blood covering the pelvic organs. Normally, your body absorbs this blood without any problems. For some reason, though, some women's bodies are unable to absorb the blood properly. The body reacts to it, causing inflammation and pain. This can lead to collections of this blood, tissue, and inflammation into aggregates called endometriosis. Endometriosis can form on the ovaries or tubes, on the outside of the uterus, on the surface of the intestines or bladder, and even rarely outside of the pelvis in the upper abdomen or chest cavity. Commonly, the implants form between the back of the uterus and the rectal wall. Ultimately, these areas turn to dense nodules and scarring, which can be very painful, especially during intercourse and bowel movements.

Endometriosis usually starts when an adolescent girl first begins menstruating. Over time, with each menstrual cycle, the symptoms worsen. Menstrual periods become a dreaded monthly battle that is painful and debilitating. If the scarring becomes severe, many women find intercourse painful or even unbearable. They can have difficulty with bowel movements or urination. Chronic pelvic pain results, affecting work, daily activities, and relationships.

In addition, endometriosis is a major cause of infertility. The exact mechanism for this association is unknown, but women with the disorder often face a difficult dilemma. They have not been able to conceive, yet they have terrible pain with each cycle. Having a hysterectomy would likely eliminate the symptoms yet leave them unable to carry a child.

Some studies suggest that endometriosis is also a risk factor for gynecologic cancers. The endometriotic implants can develop genetic mutations that lead to abnormal growth and eventually malignancies. Part of the problem is that these implants respond to hormones, particularly estrogen and progesterone. As long as the ovaries are producing these hormones, or a woman takes hormone supplements, the endometriosis is stimulated to grow and divide. For this reason, it is not advisable for some women to take hormone replacement after menopause or hysterectomy, due to the risk of stimulating their endometriosis.

Milder cases of endometriosis can be treated with medications or conservative surgery. Taking birth control pills continuously, without a week off, will sometimes control the amount of menstruation and minimize the symptoms. Anti-hormonal drugs will also block the hormonal stimulation to the endometriosis, causing the implants to regress. However, these drugs induce a temporary menopause, so the side effects of the drugs can be as bad as the endometriosis itself. Also, a young woman cannot take these medications indefinitely without long-term effects to her health. When she goes into menopause, often the symptoms will get better on their own. If excessive scarring develops, however, menopause alone won't resolve the pain.

For many women, the symptoms are so severe they cannot wait for menopause to provide relief. Surgery to remove an affected ovary or to remove implants can often resolve the problem, but these effects are sometimes only temporary. With the next few menstrual cycles, the endometriosis is back again. For these women, only a hysterectomy will help. A hysterectomy essentially gives these women their lives back for the first time in years. In very severe cases, even in young women, removing the ovaries and tubes along with the uterus is necessary to take out all of the affected tissue. Removing the ovaries also stops hormone production and therefore the hormonal stimulation to the endometriotic implants. For a young woman who has never been able to have children, having her uterus, ovaries, and tubes removed is a very emotional choice. You can imagine the amount of suffering she must have endured to arrive at this decision.

Gail, a 36-year-old married store manager, experienced difficult periods all of her life. She and her husband, who came with her to the appointment, had been trying to get pregnant for six years. She conceived twice but lost the pregnancy each time.

"I can't take the pain anymore," she told me during our office consultation. "Every month I want to curl up in a ball and die. Here are the pictures from my laparoscopy," she said, handing me the photos. "My doctor told me I'm a mess."

I looked at the pictures Gail's gynecologist had taken of her pelvic organs (via a small camera through Gail's belly button) during a recent laparoscopic procedure. Her ovaries were no longer visible, instead enveloped in reddish brown masses of old blood, glued to the back wall of her uterus. The fallopian tubes weren't identifiable either, fused somewhere in the masses. In place of nice smooth surfaces between the uterus and rectum, the rectum was welded to the back of her uterus along with the masses. I thought, *She's right. This is a mess.*

"It looks very painful," I sympathized. "How long has this been going on?"

"For years," she said. "But recently it's been much worse."

"We were still hoping for children of our own, but now we've decided to adopt." She looked at her husband and he nodded silently.

No longer trying to preserve her fertility, Gail was ready for a hysterectomy. After her robotic surgery, Gail said, "I feel like I've got my life back. Now I can just be me again."

BENIGN PELVIC MASSES

Benign ovarian tumors are sometimes treated with hysterectomy and removal of one or both of the ovaries/tubes, depending on the patient's age. In a *premenopausal* woman who wishes to maintain her fertility, an ovarian or tubal mass would not usually be treated with a hysterectomy. Instead, we would typically just remove the mass along with the tube and/or ovary to which it's attached. Preserving the remaining ovary is important to maintain hormonal function. But in a *postmenopausal* woman, since the ovaries no longer function and future pregnancy is not a concern, we generally recommend a hysterectomy with removal of both ovaries and tubes to avoid additional surgery later. The last thing we want is for these women to go through an operation for one problem and then have to come back later and have another operation for organs that aren't functioning anyway.

We introduced pelvic prolapse in the previous chapter as a symptom—the feeling of something falling out through the vagina. The word *prolapse*, though, can describe both the symptom and the condition of pelvic floor weakness. Pelvic prolapse is actually a hernia of the pelvic floor. The pelvic floor is the network of muscles that spans the distance between the bones of the pelvis and provides support for the internal organs. Injury to the pelvic floor most commonly occurs during a vaginal delivery, when the muscles and nerves are stretched and sometimes damaged as the baby comes through the birth canal. Conditions that chronically stress the pelvic floor can also lead to weakness over time. For example, overweight women are at higher risk of many kinds of hernias, including those of the pelvic floor. Their excess weight pushes down on the muscles, causing them to stretch and weaken. Chronic coughing from smoking, emphysema, or chronic bronchitis can similarly weaken the pelvic floor. When the muscles begin to lose their strength and elasticity, the internal organs of the pelvis can begin to fall through. The uterus, vagina, and intestines can all prolapse downward.

A number of non-surgical strategies exist to treat these disorders. Of course, prevention is best. Maintaining a healthy weight and avoiding smoking are the most important. However, even many fit women of a healthy weight experience prolapse later in life after having children as a younger woman.

The most common non-surgical treatment for prolapse is a pessary. The pessary, a device to hold the organs in place, fits inside the vagina like a contraceptive diaphragm. It comes in many shapes and sizes to fit different women's anatomies. Biofeedback, implantable stimulation devices, and collagen injections can also help some women with prolapse. Some cases require hysterectomy, but simply removing the uterus will not fix the pelvic defect. The most important point is to fix the hernia defect at the time of the hysterectomy. Simply removing the uterus treats the symptoms but not the condition. Without repairing the hernia defect, the other pelvic organs will eventually prolapse. In time, the bladder, vagina, and rectum can all begin to pull downward and even completely come out of the body.

In cases of prolapse, I recommend visiting a specialist in pelvic floor reconstruction such as a fellowship-trained urogynecologist.

OTHER RARE BENIGN CONDITIONS

Still other disorders are sometimes treated with hysterectomy. These include abnormalities of development of the female reproductive system, severe infections that do not respond to antibiotics, and fistulas from chronic conditions such as Crohn's disease.

PREMALIGNANT AND MALIGNANT INDICATIONS FOR HYSTERECTOMY

The word precancer is used to describe conditions where the cells of an organ have gone awry. The cells are abnormal but do not show the characteristics of cancer. We can only identify these abnormal cells by looking at them under a microscope. The most familiar test for identifying precancer is the Pap smear. When your gynecologist scrapes your cervix, she is collecting cells from both the surface and the canal of the cervix for microscopic evaluation. Pathologists examine these cells for signs of growth abnormalities. The medical word for precancer is *dysplasia*. The most important distinction between precancer and cancer is that precancers cannot invade or spread to other organs. They are therefore, by definition, not malignant. If left untreated, however, they can become cancerous over time. Identifying and treating precancer is an extremely important strategy for preventing cancer.

CERVICAL DYSPLASIA

Cervical dysplasia is caused by infection with the human papilloma virus (HPV). HPV can infect the skin and glands of the lower genital tract, including the vulva, vagina, cervix, and cervical canal. There are many different strains of the virus; some are more likely to cause genital warts while others confer a higher risk for dysplasia or cancer. Exposure to the virus occurs through sexual contact, so the more sexual partners you have, the greater the risk of exposure to a high-risk strain of HPV. However, there is more to the story than just the virus.

The vast majority of sexually active women throughout the world have been exposed to this virus with even just a few sexual partners, but most of them never develop dysplasia. There are other factors, some we know of and many others we don't, that contribute to the development of dysplasia. Essentially, all of these factors relate to a woman's immune response to the virus. For example, smoking is the most important risk factor for any HPV-related precancer or cancer. Many women do not realize that even a woman who is a non-smoker who has sex with a partner who smokes increases her risk for dysplasia. The carcinogens in cigarettes are concentrated in cervical mucus and semen, and they therefore affect the immune system's ability to fight the virus. Similarly, women who take immunosuppressive drugs for arthritis or lupus, or after an organ transplant, are at increased risk for dysplasia. And, not surprisingly, women with HIV (human immunodeficiency virus) have a weakened immune system and are at high risk for HPV-related disease.

Treatments for cervical dysplasia can be broken down into two approaches: ablative or excisional. Ablative treatments refer to *destroying* the abnormal cells, and excisional therapies refer to *removing* them. A common ablative technique includes freezing the cervix with cryotherapy. Widely used excisional procedures consist of LEEP (loop electrical excision procedure) or cervical conization. LEEP involves removing the abnormal cells with a loop-shaped wire connected to electrical cautery, while cervical conization or cone biopsy means using a surgical scalpel to remove the abnormal area. The cone biopsy gets its name from the shape of the piece of tissue removed from the cervix, which is shaped like an upside down ice cream cone. When cervical dysplasia is persistent or when high-grade dysplasia occurs in a woman no longer interested in childbearing, hysterectomy is sometimes necessary.

The most important element your surgeon must consider before performing a hysterectomy for dysplasia is to first rule out invasive cancer. If actual cancer is present, a radical hysterectomy, as opposed to a simple hysterectomy, may be necessary. A radical hysterectomy is a much more extensive operation, requiring the removal of extra tissue and lymph nodes around the cervix. If the surgeon does not know that cancer is present and performs only a simple hysterectomy instead of a radical hysterectomy, the cancer may not be properly removed. This can lead to a higher chance of the cancer coming back. Definitely *not* what we want.

ENDOMETRIAL HYPERPLASIA

This term describes overgrowth of the uterine lining. If these cells are abnormal, this condition becomes premalignant and, if left untreated, can become cancer over time. Hyperplasia typically causes abnormal bleeding. Because of the detrimental hormonal effects of obesity, being overweight is a significant risk factor for endometrial hyperplasia and ultimately endometrial cancer. Recent studies show that obese women with endometrial cancer are at a significant risk of dying from a condition related to their obesity, such as heart attack or stroke, within five years of their cancer diagnosis. Their chance of dying from their cancer is actually very small. In other words, the cancer is a warning flag that something is seriously wrong; unless a major change in health occurs, death from cardiovascular disease may be just around the corner.[1]

Endometrial hyperplasia is typically diagnosed by an endometrial biopsy or a dilation and curettage (D and C). Findings on a pelvic ultrasound can also suggest hyperplasia. Overgrowth of the uterine lining appears as a thickening on ultrasound. During a typical ultrasound, the technician will measure the thickness of the endometrial lining. An ultrasound can also detect irregularities in the shape of the endometrial lining from masses encroaching on the uterine cavity.

The most aggressive form of endometrial hyperplasia is complex hyperplasia with atypia. The term atypia indicates not only that there are too many cells (overgrowth), but also the cells themselves are abnormal (dysplastic). Studies have shown that when a biopsy identifies this condition, a uterine cancer is already present about 40 percent of

---

1   Ward KK, Shah NR, Saenz CC, McHale MT, Alvarez EA, Plaxe SC. "Cardiovascular disease is the leading cause of death among endometrial cancer patients." *Gynecologic Oncology.* 2012 Aug;126(2):176–9.

the time.[2] Therefore, unless childbearing is of the utmost importance to a woman with complex atypical hyperplasia, a hysterectomy and removal of the ovaries and tubes by a gynecologic oncologist is recommended. For preserving fertility, options for treating this condition non-surgically include progesterone treatment or placement of a progesterone-secreting IUD such as the Mirena device. These medical therapies are meant to be temporary treatments to buy some time until after pregnancy, but generally do not result in long-term cure.

PREMALIGNANT OVARIAN TUMORS

Premalignant ovarian tumors include ovarian tumors that are not overtly cancer but do contain abnormal cells. These tumors are more likely to come back than completely benign masses, but they do not metastasize. They are sometimes referred to as borderline tumors or tumors of low malignant potential. Roni Lowery, our patient from chapter 1, had a borderline ovarian tumor.

A new area of medical research involves understanding genetic predisposition to cancer. About 10 percent of all cancers are due to an inherited risk that runs in families. People who inherit a defective gene from one or both parents have an increased chance of getting the types of cancers affected by the function of that gene. We now have specific criteria for identifying families who may pass along this genetic predisposition from one generation to the next.

Many of you may have read Angelina Jolie's moving story about her decision to have her breasts removed because of an inherited BRCA mutation. Dara Marias, who wrote the foreword to this book, also faced the same decision. Women with this mutation must also choose whether or not to have their ovaries removed at a young age to lower their risk of ovarian cancer. Preventive surgery in patients with familial cancer syndromes is called "risk-reducing" surgery because it lowers their lifetime risk of ovarian cancer by about 99 percent. Why not 100 percent? Women with these mutations can still get a variant of ovarian cancer called primary peritoneal cancer. Primary peritoneal

---

2   Suh-Burgmann E, Hung YY, Armstrong MA. "Complex atypical endometrial hyperplasia: the risk of unrecognized adenocarcinoma and value of preoperative dilation and curettage." *American Journal of Obstetric Gynecololgy*. 2009 Sep;114(3):523–9.

cancers originate in the lining of the abdominal cavity, instead of the lining of the ovary. It is therefore important for all women to understand that removing the ovaries does not completely eliminate the possibility of this family of cancers. This is especially true in women with a genetic predisposition such as BRCA positivity. Primary peritoneal cancer behaves similarly to traditional ovarian cancer and is treated with the same methods.

Like Angelina Jolie and Dara Marias, in addition to risk-reducing surgery on their gynecologic organs, these women also have to decide whether to have their breasts removed. Can you imagine how difficult it must be to know that you have an almost 90 percent chance of getting breast cancer? By having your breasts removed that chance goes to about 1 percent. Would you do it? Would you have your children tested knowing each of them has a 50 percent chance of inheriting the same gene? Women who test positive for the BRCA gene face these difficult choices. We now have specific criteria for identifying families who may pass along this genetic predisposition from one generation to the next. For more information about these criteria and to see if you should be tested, visit *http://www.myriad.com* and take their hereditary cancer quiz.

MALIGNANT INDICATIONS FOR A HYSTERECTOMY

The term *malignancy* describes cells that have become so deviant that they ignore all normal interactions with their neighboring cells. They grow wild, invading nearby organs and spreading to distant ones through lymphatic channels or through the bloodstream. Ultimately, that is how cancers kill people—by invading other critical structures and choking off life.

All cancers are staged or categorized on a scale of I through IV. Stage is set at the time of diagnosis. Once it is set, it never changes; a cancer cannot be restaged. Some general rules of cancer staging apply to all cancer types. However, each type has particular criteria that define the different stages for that organ. For example, Stage I cancers are confined to the organ where they originated. Stage II cancers typically have spread to the soft tissue area next to the site of origin. Stage III represents a cancer that has spread to the next region of the body or to lymph nodes in the same region. Finally, Stage IV denotes cancers that have spread to distant organs or invaded all the way through surrounding organs. As an example, Stage I uterine cancer means the cancer is confined to the uterus. A stage II uterine cancer has spread into the cervix. For stage III, the cancer has either spread to the ovaries, pelvis, or surrounding lymph nodes. Stage IV means the cancer has spread to other organs like the lungs, bones, liver, or brain. It can also mean the cancer has grown from the uterus into the bladder or rectum. In any case, the stage correlates with the cancer prognosis, so that a higher stage cancer has a greater chance of returning and thus a worse prognosis.

Now, let's talk about the three most common gynecologic cancers treated with hysterectomy, including their risk factors, symptoms, and general treatment options.

CERVICAL CANCER

Cervical cancer is caused by HPV and can occur if severe dysplasia is left untreated. Again, not all women with HPV get dysplasia, and not all women with dysplasia get cervical cancer. Certain factors predispose women to the progression of dysplasia to cancer, including smoking, immunosuppression, poor nutrition, and an unhealthy lifestyle. In general, cervical cancer comes from precancer, so the same influences of lifestyle apply. Of course, identifying precancer and treating it is the key to preventing cervical cancer.

A Pap smear usually identifies early microscopic cervical cancers. The Pap smear cannot provide a definitive diagnosis but acts as a red flag to let your doctor know something is wrong. Often, a biopsy is the next step to investigate further. Small but visible cancers can cause abnormal bleeding, especially after intercourse. If your gynecologist sees a lesion on your cervix, she should biopsy it right away. Larger cancers of the cervix can cause heavy vaginal bleeding, a foul-smelling discharge, and pelvic pain.

UTERINE CANCER

Uterine cancers originate in either the uterine lining or the uterine muscle. *Endometrial cancer*, or cancer of the uterine lining, is the most common type of gynecologic cancer. Uterine muscle cancer, called a *uterine sarcoma*, is much rarer and tends to be more aggressive than most endometrial cancers.

Currently, medical science has identified two types of endometrial cancer. Type I endometrial cancer, the most common type, appears related to estrogen exposure, grows more slowly, and is usually curable with surgery alone. These cancers typically occur in women who suffer from "metabolic syndrome," a constellation of high-risk conditions such as obesity, diabetes, elevated cholesterol, and hypertension related to an unhealthy American lifestyle. Metabolic syndrome is found in about 35 percent of American adults. Women with these metabolic risk factors have a very high risk of heart disease, stroke, and metabolically related cancers such as Type I endometrial cancer. These cancers often arise in the uterine lining in a background of endometrial hyperplasia. If left untreated, the precancer cells ultimately become cancer cells.

Type II endometrial cancers are genetically distinct from Type I cancers. We find them more commonly in older, thinner women. They have a more aggressive behavior pattern and grow in an otherwise normal or even dormant uterine lining. In general, treatment for Type II cancers involves a combination of surgery, chemotherapy, and radiation.

Uterine cancers are staged based on the findings at the time of surgery. Therefore, the stage of any woman's uterine cancer is not known until the surgery is performed and all the removed tissue is analyzed by the pathology laboratory. It can take several days to a week to receive a final report. A total hysterectomy (uterus and cervix) and removal of the ovaries/tubes is the minimum surgery in all cases. In many situations, additional removal of surrounding lymph nodes is necessary to look for spread of abnormal cells. In a smaller number of cases, usually for the more aggressive Type II cancers, removal of other abdominal tissues can help identify other areas of spread.

Uterine sarcomas evolve from the muscular wall of the uterus. Uterine fibroids also arise from the uterine muscle but are benign. Many women with fibroids are afraid their fibroids will "turn to cancer," but this just doesn't happen. However, the *symptoms* of fibroids and sarcomas overlap. In both cases, the uterus becomes enlarged from a mass, and abnormal bleeding is common. Nobody knows exactly what causes sarcomas, but women with a prior history of pelvic radiation have an increased risk of uterine sarcoma.

OVARIAN CANCER

Known as the "silent killer," ovarian cancer can sneak up on a woman with vague symptoms that mimic other common benign conditions. Abdominal or pelvic discomfort, urinary urgency, constipation, and pelvic fullness are common. But these same symptoms can occur from something as innocuous as a urinary tract infection or as common as diverticulitis. However, in the case of ovarian cancer, the symptoms worsen and progress to abdominal bloating and the inability to eat. At this point, most women realize something is wrong, but unfortunately, the cancer is likely to be advanced already.

To make matters scarier, currently there is NO screening test for ovarian cancer. Many women are confused by inaccurate recommendations they might read in women's magazines. I have seen articles suggesting that all women should demand from their doctor a CA-125 blood test to "check for ovarian cancer." Unfortunately, the CA-125 test is not accurate in the capacity of a screening test. For that to be the case, a CA-125 value, if checked on a normal healthy woman, would be able to distinguish between a woman who does or does not have ovarian cancer. However, about one-third of women with ovarian cancer have a normal CA-125. In addition, as we've discussed, many other conditions make the CA-125 abnormal, such as appendicitis, endometriosis, fibroids, cirrhosis of the liver, pelvic inflammation, recent surgery, ectopic pregnancy, etc. Since the test can't distinguish between cancer and non-cancer, it is not useful to screen all women. However, it *is* used as a marker to track the progress of treatment in a woman with known ovarian cancer. As I discussed in the section on pelvic masses, it can also be used in a woman with a mass to give some indication, prior to surgery, whether the mass is likely to be benign or malignant. That's why Roni Lowery's doctor ordered one for her. However, for the reasons mentioned, it is only a general guide and doesn't reliably "diagnose" cancer preoperatively. Along the same lines, when a woman with a mass has a normal CA-125, it doesn't mean she doesn't have cancer. Only by surgically removing the mass can we be sure. When Roni's test results were abnormal, it certainly made her even more anxious about what might be wrong with her.

Sometimes ovarian cancer cannot be diagnosed until the time of surgery. But, in many cases, all the signs point to it.

When I first met Linda, sitting in a chair across from me at our consultation table, she looked sick. Her skin was pale, her face gaunt, and her eyes sunken. Her belly was hugely swollen.

"About four months ago, I started having pain right here," she told me, pointing to her bladder. "I went to my family doctor, and he treated me for a urinary tract infection. But the pain got worse."

I asked her if she was having any trouble moving her bowels or urinating. "Yes," she admitted. "I only pee a little bit at a time, and I've been constipated for months. Normally I am pretty regular."

Linda pointed to her belly and told me, "My stomach started to swell about a month ago. The last few weeks, I can hardly eat more than a few bites."

I examined her and felt a large, irregular mass stuck in her pelvis and pushing against her rectum. Her stomach was tensely swollen with fluid.

Her CT scan showed a large mass in her pelvis and other masses near her stomach. A large amount of abnormal fluid surrounded her abdominal organs. Her CA-125 test was over 4,000 units/mL.

Linda knew her situation was grave, but her biggest concern was whether she would be able to care for her mother, who suffered from dementia. Not wanting to shy away from the obvious, I looked her in the eye. "Right now, we have to focus on taking care of *you*. If you're not around, who will take care of your mother?"

Linda nodded and said, "I'll do whatever I can to get better."

Ovarian cancer affects about 1 in 70 women over their lifetime. To put this in perspective, about 1 in 8 women will get breast cancer. But, although ovarian cancer is uncommon, it is devastating when it does occur. Treatment typically involves both surgery and chemotherapy. Surgery for early ovarian cancer has two goals: diagnose the cancer and identify its stage. For advanced cases, the goals shift:

diagnose the cancer and remove all involved areas that can safely be extracted. Like uterine cancers, ovarian cancers are staged based on the findings at the time of surgery, so the cancer stage cannot be known until comprehensive surgical staging/debulking (removal of the tumor) is performed.

Standard surgical staging procedures for ovarian cancer include hysterectomy with bilateral salpingo-oophorectomy (BSO: both ovaries and tubes), an omentectomy, removal of pelvic and abdominal lymph nodes, and biopsies of the abdominal cavity. The omentum is a large fatty internal apron of tissue that drapes off the colon and stomach.

Ovarian cancers commonly spread to this organ, and it should be removed in all ovarian cancer surgery. Debulking surgery for more advanced disease also includes hysterectomy/BSO, but often much more than that. Omentectomy, removal of diseased areas on the intestines, colon, diaphragm, liver, or spleen may also be necessary. In debulking surgery, essentially any area that is involved needs to be removed if surgically feasible. The goal of ovarian cancer debulking surgery is to complete the operation with the minimum of visible cancer remaining because chemotherapy is always necessary after surgery for advanced ovarian cancer, and the treatments are most effective when beginning with the smallest number of cancer cells left behind to treat.

NON-GYNECOLOGIC CANCERS

Cancers originating in other organs of the body occasionally spread to the female reproductive system. Breast and colorectal cancer are the most common types we see, but even cancers of the lung, pancreas, stomach, lymph cells (lymphomas), and others can metastasize to the uterus, ovaries, and tubes. In these situations, the cancer may have also spread to other organs as well, and removing the female organs may not improve survival. However, if the metastasis is causing symptoms, there are some situations where hysterectomy may improve quality of life.

. . .

This brief overview gave you a glimpse into the complexity of the many gynecologic problems that can lead a woman to seek hysterectomy. The thought of having a serious condition such as cancer or needing a hysterectomy can be frightening. But addressing those fears gives you the best opportunity for good health. If you have any of the symptoms or conditions we've discussed, the most important step you can take is to discuss your health history and options with your doctor to find out what's right for you. Since these conversations are so important, I have dedicated the next chapter to helping you prepare for them with confidence.

Chapter 6

WHAT YOU SHOULD KNOW ABOUT YOUR DOCTOR AND WHAT SHE SHOULD KNOW ABOUT YOU

In your hysterectomy story, the most important players are you and your surgeon. Remember, not all surgeons are created equal. Some gynecologists excel in the delivery room, while others showcase their skills in the operating room. We all have innate talents that give us natural abilities for certain types of work. However, like any other profession, we also differ in our motivation and drive to excel and improve. Some work harder than others to hone their skills.

Training programs differ markedly from each other around the country and around the world. Some programs emphasize innovation in the operating room, others in the laboratory. Severe limitations on work hours are now mandated for doctors-in-training. This affects the number of cases they have performed at the time of graduation, and many programs struggle to provide an adequate surgical experience to their graduates.

In addition, surgeons discover their own biases and tendencies as they begin to practice. It is important to understand that these biases affect their recommendations when they see you as a patient. For example, although I am skilled in performing all types of hysterectomy surgeries, I'm biased toward minimally invasive surgery (MIS) and more specifically toward robotic surgery. I simply believe it's better, when appropriate, both for my patients and for me as their surgeon.

Surgeons are trained to create routines. At first, we learn the routines of our teachers. As we gain confidence and experience, we modify those routines, perhaps taking a method from one teacher and blending it with a technique from another. Once we learn a routine, we want to follow it the same way every time. In my own experience, once I've established a successful pattern of doing some task, I tend to repeat that routine regularly. That way, I am more likely to proceed through those series of moves more efficiently and am less likely to forget something. At the same time, surgeons want to balance routine with creativity, because innovation leads to improvements in the future. I try regularly to identify areas where I am less than completely satisfied with my approach and constantly tweak my routine to achieve greater efficiency. My desire to improve and grow as a surgeon led me to learn robotic surgery in the first place.

Mastering laparoscopy requires skills over and above those needed to be proficient at open surgery. The surgeon must have an exceptional understanding of anatomy, as well as the dexterity to perform the surgical movements. The surgeon must also possess the ability to think in 3-D, superimposing a mental image of her anatomical knowledge onto the case at hand. She must use both hands simultaneously. For example, the left hand retracts the bladder while the right hand dissects it from the uterus. I believe some people possess an innate talent for these skills, but any craft improves with practice and hard work.

A doctor who trained at an institution well known for a certain type of procedure will probably gain a great deal of experience with that particular procedure. In practice, her tendency will be to treat most of her patients with that same familiar procedure. A broad surgical experience means she can recommend the best procedure from a list of many that she knows well. A good analogy is the toolbox of a car mechanic. When your car needs service, you bring it to a mechanic with the tools available to diagnose and fix the problem. Nowadays, most good repair shops have a full array of wrenches, nut drivers, and pliers, but they also have air compressors, hydraulic lifts, and computer diagnostics. If you went to a shop that didn't have some of these items, but they still wanted your business, they might suggest the fix they have, not necessarily the fix that's best.

My advice is this: research your doctor. If she is competent, she should welcome your questions about her skill and experience. Remember Roni Lowery, the patient featured at the start of this book? Her most important message is to feel confident in your doctor. Not only should you feel confident in her abilities, but also in her understanding of your needs as a unique individual. In most cases, patients go to a surgeon via a referral from another physician. A good recommendation by your primary doctor reflects back on them. Doctors who have worked in a community for a while usually know the other specialists well and can attest to the quality of their work. When I refer one of my own patients to a specialist in a different field, I look for someone who is well trained, current with new medical knowledge, skilled, and compassionate. I also value a low complication rate and good judgment in dealing with complications. Be aware, however, that some doctors refer patients for reasons other than quality.

They may only refer within a specific social network or based on the number of referrals back to them. Sometimes, an insurance network mandates a referral to a specific doctor. Therefore, don't completely rely on a referral from another doctor. Do some inquiry yourself.

To help you through this inquiry process, the reference section at the end of this book provides a list of suggested questions to ask your surgeon.

The first area to address in your inquiry is background and training. You can contact the doctor's office for this information or research her online. Many practices provide biographical summaries of their doctors on their websites. As a minimum requirement, ask your doctor if she is board certified in obstetrics and gynecology. If she is a gynecologic oncologist, ask if she also has subspecialty board certification in gynecologic oncology. This board certification signifies that the doctor has achieved a standard level of knowledge and competence as designated by a group of leaders in each specific field. To become board certified in obstetrics and gynecology, a physician must pass a series of milestones. First, she must successfully complete a four-year, board-approved residency program. Within three years of completion, she must pass a written examination. Then she is eligible to begin collecting a case list of patients cared for during a one-year period. The physician then sits for an oral examination covering theoretical questions and questions about patients on the list. After passing all examinations, the doctor receives a diploma of board certification, which must be updated annually. The process for subspecialty certification in gynecologic oncology involves all of those steps, with the addition of the following extra achievements. After completing a four-year residency and being accepted into a board-accredited program, a gynecologic oncologist must successfully complete a three- or four-year fellowship in gynecologic oncology. The physician must pass the written and oral exams for general obstetrics and gynecology and then begin the process all over again for the subspecialty boards in gynecologic oncology. There is a written examination, testing knowledge in the field. Then the physician collects a new case list of patients cared for over a period of one year. During the oral examination, she must defend the case list and a research thesis, and she must answer theoretical patient management questions. As you can see, the process of board certification ensures that practicing physicians have achieved an appropriate baseline level of competence. Asking your doctor about her certification status ensures that she has met that standard before she operates on you.

You also may want to know something about the doctor's practice structure. For example, in some groups, the doctor you see in the office may not be the doctor who actually does your surgery. One of the other partners in the group could be assigned to your case. I certainly recommend that the surgeon you meet with in the office—the one who discussed all the particulars of your case with you, the one who listened to your concerns and needs, the one who examined you—is the same one who actually does your surgery.

Some practices work with residents and fellows—that is, surgeons-in-training. There are pros and cons to this arrangement. Academic centers can sometimes offer treatments that are not available through private practitioners. Having young and eager minds attentive to your case can spark innovative approaches. However, some patients are not comfortable with a surgeon-in-training performing their operation, so do understand this trade-off when seeking care with practices that participate in training programs. Find out how the residents are supervised and what level of involvement they will have in your operation and after-care.

To complete your inquiry about your doctor's background, find out where she trained. You may not have heard of her institution or program, but going through her educational history should give you a feeling of confidence, not concern.

The next portion of your assessment deals with experience and judgment and can usually only be discovered during an in-person meeting. Whichever method of hysterectomy is recommended, ask her how many cases like yours she has done. Be aware that published guidelines do not exist for how much surgery is enough surgery. One study from New York found that surgeons who perform fewer than 10 hysterectomies per year were more likely to perform those surgeries with an open incision, or a total abdominal hysterectomy (TAH). Busier surgeons were more likely to utilize alternative, less invasive techniques.[3] Other studies set the bar at 30 hysterectomy cases per year to distinguish high volume surgeons from low volume surgeons.[4] As a comparison, I perform about 175 hysterectomies per year, out of about 375 cases annually, including non-hysterectomy cases.

Next, find out what selection criteria your doctor uses in deciding what method of surgery to recommend. Criteria such as your age, weight, uterine size, indication for hysterectomy, and previous surgical history might affect this recommendation. One of the key messages I hope you will take away from this book is to explore whether you are a candidate for minimally invasive or robotic surgery.

Robotic surgery requires special training and development of new skills. If you are a candidate for robotic surgery, you want to explore your surgeon's robotic experience. How many robotic cases has she done, and more importantly, what is her surgical volume per week, per month, and per year? With any method of MIS, the rate of *conversion* should be explored. When a case is started laparoscopically but the surgeon is unable to complete it without opening the abdomen, we call that a conversion. This may be required when the disease process is more complex than anticipated and cannot be safely addressed laparoscopically. Conversion may also be necessary to deal with a complication such as bleeding or injury. A surgeon's conversion rate is an excellent indicator of her overall proficiency and judgment. Therefore, if MIS is considered, ask about her conversion rate. About two to five percent is an acceptable rate typically reported in the medical literature.[5] A rate higher than that should be cause for concern. If your doctor says she never has a conversion, she either is hiding something or doesn't do enough surgery to encounter the need for conversion. As with all complications, surgeons always try to

---

3   Boyd LR, Novetsky AP, Curtin JP. "Effect of surgical volume on route of hysterectomy and short-term morbidity." *American Journal of Obstetric Gynecology.* 2010 Oct;116(4):909–15.

4   Worley MJ Jr, Anwandter C, Sun CC, dos Reis R, Nick AM, Frumovitz M, Soliman PT, Schmeler KM, Levenback CF, Munsell MF, Ramirez PT. "Impact of surgeon volume on patient safety in laparoscopic gynecologic surgery." *Gynecologic Oncology.* 2012 Apr;125(1):241–4.

5   Paley PJ, Veljovich DS, Shah CA, Everett EN, Bondurant AE, Drescher CW, Peters WA 3rd. "Surgical outcomes in gynecologic oncology in the era of robotics: analysis of first 1000 cases." *American Journal of Obstetric Gynecology.* 2011 Jun;204(6):551.e1–9.

avoid them. However, over the career of even the best surgeon, some complications are inevitable. A surgeon with occasional complications is NOT cause for alarm, nor is it a sign of a bad doctor. The most important issue is how the surgeon handles those complications. You want a surgeon who realistically tracks her own complication rate and critically assesses the root cause of each one. Forthright self-assessment is a sign of confidence and good judgment.

• • •

Up until now, we've been talking about how to get to know your doctor, but, of course, your doctor needs to know quite a bit about you. To care for you thoroughly, your doctor needs certain key pieces of information about your health history, your current health status, and your individual desires and concerns. When I see patients in my practice, I approach each one like a puzzle. Part of my job is to find the important pieces of the puzzle and put them together to create an accurate portrait of that individual. In other words, you are most likely to have a safe and successful outcome if you go see your doctor prepared with all the information she will need. Your doctor will want to know all the pieces of your unique history so she can develop a picture of you. We can break these pieces down into four main groups:

- The information you need to fill out your health questionnaire
- Your past medical records
- Details about your current problem
- Your feelings regarding important issues related to your surgery

Let's walk through these steps together to get you ready for your appointment. (In the reference section in the back of this book, I include a handy list of things you need to prepare for your visit. Of course, your doctor may request additional information, but this should cover the majority of important areas.)

First, be prepared to fill out a number of forms that review your health history. Although these questionnaires are often time consuming, they are not meant to be a burden. Instead, they are an important way for your doctor to learn as much about you as possible.

TECHNICAL DETOUR: BONUS READING MATERIAL

Does your surgeon look at her specimens in the operating room with the pathologist?

Presumably, doctors perform hysterectomies because something is wrong with the female organs. Ultimately, surgeons must rely on pathologists to analyze the organs we remove and provide us with a final diagnosis. Proper handling of pathology specimens ensures a quality report that provides the information we need to treat our patients.

In the operating room, once the surgeon removes a part of the body, she will tell the staff how she wants the specimen labeled and processed. During a hysterectomy, the surgeon typically hands the uterus off the sterile area to a nurse who is not scrubbed in. The surgeon must verbally describe the specimen to document what was removed. A common example would be "TLH/BSO" or total laparoscopic hysterectomy and bilateral salpingo-oophorectomy. Then the surgeon informs the staff how she would like the specimen processed. She typically chooses one of the following three methods:

1. Open the uterus, ovaries, and tubes to examine the lining with the naked eye.

2. Place the specimen in a formalin container for later examination by the pathologist.

3. Ask the pathologist to perform an immediate preliminary analysis, called a frozen section, on any mass or suspicious areas in the uterus, ovaries, or tubes.

Certainly, in any case where cancer is even a possibility, *someone*—the surgeon or the pathologist—should look at what's just been removed. Remember that until the uterus is opened, we can't really know what's inside of it. I like to see the uterine lining and muscular wall of just about every case with my own eyes. If an abnormality is identified, a frozen section can be performed while the patient is still asleep. Frozen section refers to the procedure where the pathologist takes a small portion of a mass or organ, freezes it in liquid nitrogen, and then looks at it under the microscope. In most cases, the frozen section gives a very accurate preliminary examination of the removed tissue. If cancer is found, the surgeon can act on those

findings immediately, during the operation. The alternative means waiting several days for the pathology report. By that time, the patient may have already gone home and may have to return for another operation.

In my opinion, the best approach is to discuss each case personally with the pathologist. Good communication between doctors fosters better patient care and positive working relationships. In addition, it's important that the pathologist know what the surgeon expects from their analysis. In most cases these days, the pathologist is not the one who prepares the specimen for microscopic examination. This is usually done by a technician, who may not be familiar with the treatment of gynecologic conditions. For all these reasons, I recommend asking your surgeon if she will be looking at your specimen with the pathologist during your hysterectomy. If this habit is not part of her regular routine, consider finding another surgeon.

Here are two examples to illustrate my point. First, let's review the case of Betty. She was 64 years old, with postmenopausal bleeding. We were unable to perform an endometrial biopsy or D and C because the opening to her cervix was scarred. When I did her hysterectomy and BSO, the pathologist opened the uterus and found a large cancer inside. I completed the surgical staging right then by removing pelvic and abdominal lymph nodes.

Another example is that of Marjorie. She was a 42-year-old mother of four who suffered from abnormal bleeding. An endometrial biopsy was normal, and the bleeding was thought to be from fibroids. She wanted to retain her ovaries to preserve her hormones but needed the hysterectomy to stop the bleeding. In the operating room, we opened the uterus and found an unusual mass in the uterine wall. The frozen section showed a sarcoma, a cancer of the muscular wall of the uterus. We removed the ovaries and tubes because leaving them behind could compromise her chance of cure from her cancer. Without the frozen section, we would have had to bring her back for another operation to remove the ovaries/tubes and complete the cancer staging.

In my practice, forms can be downloaded from our website, so patients can fill them out at home. This can be a real time-saver at your office visit, and many practices now provide this service. Some patients fill out their forms on their computer and bring in a printed copy. This is ideal, because the forms are usually more complete and legible.

When you sit down to fill out these forms, focus on some key areas. Once you get past the obvious demographic questions, such as your age, address, phone numbers, etc., you will get to a section about your past medical history. When I look at this section as a surgeon, I'm looking for a list of any medical conditions you have been diagnosed with at any time in your life. Examples would be disorders like high blood pressure, diabetes, lupus, heart disease, kidney stones, low thyroid, etc. Any of these conditions could be relevant to your current problem and could affect your surgery.

Next on the list is your past surgical history. Record any operation or procedure you have had in your life, even if it was many years ago. You may not know it, but that colon surgery you had 10 years ago may be tremendously important to your surgeon today. If you have any records from past surgeries, bring them with you to your visit. The key documents surgeons want to see are the operative report and the pathology report. The operative report is the surgeon's dictated account of the operation. It states what was done, how it was done, and any relevant findings. The pathology report is the description of what was taken out and what it looked like under the microscope. The operative report states what parts were removed and how they were removed, while the pathology report shows what was wrong with them. Often, the search to acquire old medical records causes more delays in diagnosis and treatment of a current problem more than any other obstacle to surgery. When I see my patients for their first post-operative visit, I give them a copy of these reports for their records.

Bring a list of all your medications and supplements, including dosages. Include a list of any medical allergies. Even allergies to tape, certain kinds of soap, or intravenous dye are important information. If you have a problem with certain types of medication like pain pills, include this information. I often ask patients if they have taken particular narcotics, like Percocet® or Lortab® in the past. If a medicine was beneficial before, that lets me know it will probably be a good choice again.

Additionally, try to sketch a brief history of your family's health, especially noting any close relatives with cancer. Your doctor will want to know what kind of cancer they had, at what age, and their current health status. Other medical problems that run in your family could also be important. For example, some patients tell me that all the women in their family have needed a hysterectomy for fibroids. Others report a family history of anesthesia complications.

A section on your lifestyle is next on our list. This includes smoking history, use of recreational drugs, and alcohol consumption. Doctors need to know how much you smoke and for how many years. Even if you are not a smoker, let your doctor know if you have significant exposure to secondhand smoke. Be honest. Smoking is a risk factor for many reproductive problems such as cervical precancer, cervical cancer, vulvar precancer, vulvar cancer, vaginal precancer, vaginal cancer, and pelvic prolapse. Also, use of drugs and alcohol can predispose you to certain reactions after surgery and are important to disclose. Some patients are embarrassed to disclose how much they smoke or whether they use drugs or alcohol. Your doctor is not there to judge you but to help you, so be honest about your habits.

Now that we have covered filling out all your forms, what's next? Gather copies of any relevant medical tests you may have had. This may require multiple phone calls or trips to the facilities where these tests were done, including ultrasounds, CT scans, MRI scans, PET scans, etc. Many people don't realize that these reports may not be readily available to your doctor. Never assume that any of your doctors have a complete record of all your health care history. Currently, medical care is very compartmentalized. You go to one doctor for your heart, another for your eyes, and your gynecologist for your reproductive organs. (Congress passed the HITECH act in 2009. This law mandates that all physicians computerize their medical records; however, there are dozens of different types of software, and none of those systems talk to each other.) Doctors often still have to rely on faxing reports to one another. The best way to ensure that all your records are kept in one place is to keep them yourself.

When it comes to imaging studies, there is a difference between a scan *report* and the actual scan. The report is the dictated analysis from the radiologist who read the scan. The images are the actual pictures of your body that the radiologist looks at to compose the report. Traditionally, these were printed on large sheets of x-ray film and then placed in paper jackets. Nowadays, the images are digitized, so they are commonly saved to a disc or flash drive. Many doctors, including me, like to look at the actual images from CTs or MRIs. I ask my patients to bring copies of both the report and the scan to their office visit. You can get copies from the radiology facility where the scan was performed.

Also bring in a copy of any pathology reports related to your current medical condition. Recent Pap smears and any biopsy reports are most critical. If you had a biopsy done, such as an office endometrial biopsy or a dilation and curettage, make sure you get a copy of the results. If you need to see another physician for the same problem, this piece of information may be key to receiving the best medical treatment.

The next area to prepare for is how you explain your problem to the doctor. Generally, she will want to know what your current symptoms are, how long they have been going on, and any treatments you may have tried to treat them. What activities affect the symptoms? Do your menstrual cycles have any impact on the problem? Have you noticed any recent changes in your bowel or bladder habits? Did the symptoms come on gradually or all at once? All of this information is important to understand your condition.

Many women come to me expecting a consultation without a physical exam, which I find surprising. Never let a doctor operate on you without examining you first, except in an emergency setting. A consultation always includes a physical examination; otherwise, how can we offer an opinion about your condition? Believe me, as a woman, I know that no one likes a pelvic exam. But, just as your cardiologist has to listen to your heart and your ophthalmologist has to look in your eyes, your gynecologist has to examine your reproductive organs. Very often, this is the time during the consultation when I plan the operation in my mind—if that's what I think is needed. I am considering all the pieces of the puzzle, plugging them into my

Surgeon's Logic and coming up with a treatment plan that I think will best suit the patient. No matter how fancy CT scans, PET scans, and other medical technology becomes, there is still no substitute for a skilled doctor touching the patient with her own hands.

Most women don't realize that the rectal exam is often the most important part of the pelvic. Why? Because the doctor can best feel the pelvic organs on the rectal exam. For women under 30, women without a premalignant or malignant condition, or without a history of cancer in the family, the rectal exam can sometimes be omitted. However, the rectal is recommended as a routine in ANY woman over 40 to screen for anorectal cancer. These cancers are common, and an exam is a simple way to check this area during a routine physical. In the near future, your doctor will be able to smear her finger on a card after the rectal to check for abnormal DNA in your stool. This test will be an accurate means to pick up colorectal cancer or precancer. It may seem strange to you, but *ask* for the rectal exam. If you meet the criteria I just mentioned and aren't getting one, this may warn you of a doctor who is less than thorough.

Finally, be prepared to talk to your doctor about your feelings and desires. How your hysterectomy story unfolds depends a great deal on how honest you are with your doctor about your fears and feelings. When you need a hysterectomy, it's normal to worry about how the surgery will affect you. Are you hoping to have children in the future? How do you feel about menopause? Are you afraid of your future risk of cancer? Are you concerned about the possibility of needing surgery in the future? Is the appearance of any scar(s) important to you? What type of work do you do? Do you exercise regularly? Are you sexually active? Who will take care of you while you recover from surgery? Who will help take care of your household while you recover? These are all important questions that may directly affect how your surgery proceeds.

Share your feelings with your doctor. Remember that trust Roni Lowery was looking for in her surgeon? That feeling that the surgeon would do what was best for her no matter what? That's how you should feel about your surgeon by the end of your visit. Your doctor has to earn that trust by sharing her compassion and expertise with you.

Surgeons have many choices today about how to accomplish a hysterectomy. But no matter how your hysterectomy is performed, your anatomy, your medical condition, your individual circumstances, and basic surgical principles dictate the steps of the operation. As you will see, the way your surgeon accomplishes each step varies greatly from one method to another. To understand the different methods is to understand the evolution of the modern hysterectomy. Let's take a look at how we got where we are today.

Chapter 7

NOT ALL HYSTERECTOMIES ARE CREATED EQUAL:
THE TALE OF THE MODERN HYSTERECTOMY

This is the story of an operation that traditionally marked the transition from mother to matron, from youth to old age, from possibility to past tense. If we trace the history of the hysterectomy, we'll find it parallels the history of a woman's place in the modern medical establishment. Over the years, women have gained a sense of control of our bodies. We know that our medical choices affect our careers, our families, and our feelings of self-worth. We want better outcomes with fewer harmful side effects. We want to be healthy and productive, and we want a say in how our medical care keeps us that way. The evolution of the modern hysterectomy, in essence, mirrors the evolution of the modern woman.

This story starts in ancient times, when women rarely survived early attempts at emergency hysterectomy. Vaginal hysterectomies were first performed safely in the 1800s, but even today, this approach is limited to treating simpler gynecologic problems. Over a hundred years ago, the first abdominal hysterectomies were performed for complex conditions. These early abdominal operations were dangerous and disfiguring. Improvements in anesthesia and antibiotics made things safer but not less invasive. Women felt embarrassed to talk about their bodies in those times. Hysterectomy resulted in feeling a loss of femininity, as if one's very womanhood was being taken away. Large incisions on the abdomen allowed the surgeon's hands to manipulate the organs directly, but with all the attendant effects on body image and overall health. In the 1980s, laparoscopic surgery entered the picture. By putting scopes into the belly instead of our hands, we turned our eyes toward the deeper impact surgical techniques have on our patients. A picture of new possibilities came into focus. Women had less pain, shorter recoveries, and less time off from work and family. But the women with the most to gain from these new procedures were still shut out due to limitations in technology. In 2005, robotic surgery was introduced to gynecology, opening up access for many women to experience surgery without the suffering.

In the current era, we have six methods for performing a basic hysterectomy. These six methods include:

- Total abdominal hysterectomy (TAH)
- Total vaginal hysterectomy (TVH)

- Laparoscopically-assisted vaginal hysterectomy (LAVH)
- Total laparoscopic hysterectomy (TLH)
- Supracervical hysterectomy (SH)
- Robotic hysterectomy (RH)

I will also briefly discuss a special type of hysterectomy, the radical hysterectomy, used only for cervical cancer treatment.

In chapter 5, "So You Think You Need a Hysterectomy: The Why behind Your Operation," we discussed the typical diseases requiring hysterectomy, such as fibroids, prolapse, endometriosis, benign tumors, precancer, or cancer. When these conditions become life threatening or severely limiting to a woman's quality of life, a hysterectomy becomes necessary. Although the reason for the operation may be different from one woman to another, all methods share the same essential steps required for removal of the uterus. The primary distinction between the methods is the access. What I mean by access is the type of incision the surgeon uses to gain entrance to the body to remove the uterus. How is one method different from another? Let's explore this further.

TOTAL ABDOMINAL HYSTERECTOMY (TAH): THE OLD STANDARD

Since the mid-1800s, the TAH (or open hysterectomy) has been the standard operation for removing the uterus. This is the operation our mothers faced in previous generations, and ultimately, all methods of hysterectomy are derived from it. The steps to performing a TAH follow a classic script that all gynecologists learn in their training, with these moves so ingrained in us during residency that they become as routine as tying our shoes. We learn the mantra "Clamp, cut, suture" until we can repeat it in our sleep!

The first stage of any operation involves anesthetizing, prepping, and draping the patient. The thoughtful surgeon is involved every step of the way, making sure there is good communication between all members of the surgical team to achieve a good outcome. After making the incision, we use a retractor to hold the sides of the incision open. We carefully pack sponges into the abdomen to hold the intestines out of the way and establish a clear view of the reproductive organs. Then we can begin the actual removal of the uterus. Here is the step-by-step process:

1. Clamp along the sides of the uterus to provide traction.
2. If we are removing the ovaries, clamp, cut, and suture (stitch) the blood vessels going to them.
3. If we are leaving the ovaries, clamp, cut, and suture the blood vessels between the uterus and ovaries, leaving the ovarian vessels intact.
4. Divide the ligaments holding the sides of the uterus.
5. Separate the tissues between the bladder and the cervix so that the bladder is out of harm's way.
6. Isolate the uterine arteries. Clamp, cut, and suture them.
7. Clamp, cut, and suture the tissues and blood vessels next to the cervix.
8. Clamp, cut, and suture the ligaments on the back of the uterus.
9. Clamp the vagina on either side.
10. Separate the uterus and cervix where they attach to the vagina.
11. Suture the vaginal cuff where the uterus and cervix were separated from the top of the vagina.

Refer back to figure 2 from "Anatomy 101." This diagram shows how the ureter courses right through the uterine vessels, making this area prone to injury during a hysterectomy. The purpose of step 1, putting traction on the uterus, pulls it away from the bladder, rectum, and ureters, lowering the risk of injury.

The next few steps involve separating the uterus from its surrounding tissues. In step 5, we move the bladder away before the uterus and cervix can be safely separated from the top of the vagina; otherwise, the bladder could be cut, too. The next steps involve controlling the uterine blood supply. Then in step 10, the uterus and cervix are separated from where they meet the vagina, and they are removed from the body. Finally, in step 11, the upper part of the vagina is sewn together with dissolving suture so the area can heal smoothly.

These steps are the foundation of any hysterectomy, after which the surgeon checks everything, removes the sponges and retractor, and closes the incision with stitches.

For the surgeon, advantages of the TAH primarily relate to being able to see and feel. Keeping the intestines or other organs packed away from the surgical area is most reliable with the open technique because large retractors and sponge packs can be placed to achieve a clear view. Also, with an open incision, all the nooks and crannies of the abdominal cavity can be felt. This is particularly important in an advanced cancer case, when all areas of the abdomen must be checked. Especially for ovarian cancer, when small tumor nodules can grow on any surface of the abdominal organs, there is no substitute for the tactile awareness of the human hand.

The TAH has saved thousands of lives over the years, but there are many disadvantages to the operation. Remember Fran Lowery, Roni's mother? When she had her TAH, she suffered through a great deal of pain and a fear of burdening her husband during her recovery. Worse yet, her incision opened up a few weeks after surgery, prolonging the healing process even further. That is one of the risks of a large incision. Even if the appearance of the scar is not important to you, what happens on the inside should be. The body must go through a healing process when recovering from any surgery. Healing requires more of your energy and bodily resources when the surgery is more invasive.

Within the first few hours after incision, a reaction to the trauma of surgery begins. The body sends inflammatory cells to the injured tissue, creating pain and swelling. The more invasive the surgery, the more the body loses blood and fluid because of trauma to a larger area. Bacteria can enter the injured area, eventually leading to infection if not contained by the body's immune mechanisms. The intestines become swollen and inactive, not performing their normal movements to propel food through the system. This explains why many people don't have an appetite after abdominal surgery. Finally, surgery hurts. When you have pain, you don't move around or take deep breaths well. Inactivity can cause stagnant blood and blood clots. Shallow breathing increases the risk of pneumonia. Also, the stress of surgery becomes a limiting factor in patients who are elderly or who have other medical problems like a weak heart, arthritis, or diabetes.

Once the body has recovered from the initial shock of surgical trauma, the healing process begins. Unfortunately, part of healing involves scarring. Internal scarring can lead to adhesions, whereby organs that are not normally attached become welded together with bands of tissue. The effects of adhesions depend on where they occur. For example, adhesions involving the intestines can lead to pain with bowel movements, cramping, or even bowel blockages. Adhesions around the pelvic structures can lead to pain with urination, generalized pain, or pain with intercourse. Adhesions around the ovaries can lead to pain with ovulation.

Other problems with healing can involve the scar itself. The abdominal wall is made of many layers, all of which have to heal together after being cut open. Sometimes, especially if infection sets in, the deep layers of the wound can come open completely, requiring emergency surgery. A skin separation, although not an emergency, is very distressing for the patient. An open wound is scary and painful. Extended periods of wound care, usually administered by home health nurses, is required for ultimate healing. Once the scar eventually heals, it is typically wider and more unsightly.

Certain patients are at much higher risk of these complications than others are. Diabetes impairs wound healing and increases susceptibility to infection. Obesity is a major risk factor for a wound complication. A thicker abdominal wall creates a friendly environment for bacterial growth and infection, and the physical weight of a heavier abdomen can pull the incision apart. In addition, the same operation must be performed through a larger incision on an obese patient than on a thin patient. This larger incision is needed because it is more difficult to see critical structures when the abdominal wall is thicker.

Strategies to minimize the trauma of surgery are key to improving patient outcomes. Of course, the use of antibiotics lowers the risk of infection. Adhesion barriers decrease the severity of scar tissue formation. Narcotics help patients cope with the pain of surgical recovery. Newer surgical retractors may decrease trauma to the skin and abdominal wall. However, no matter how we try to compensate, the bottom line is this: the larger the incision, the more profound the stress response to the trauma of surgery. The TAH was Fran Lowery's hysterectomy, and more than likely, it was your mother's hysterectomy too—but it doesn't have to be yours.

TOTAL VAGINAL HYSTERECTOMY (TVH): THE ORIGINAL MINIMALLY INVASIVE HYSTERECTOMY

For almost two hundred years, surgeons have performed hysterectomies without scars by performing the entire operation through the vagina. The key term here is THROUGH the vagina. This means the surgeon's view is through the vagina, the instruments are used through the vagina, and the access to all the reproductive organs is through the vagina. This is important because the access is limited by the narrow width of the vaginal canal. Although feeling is preserved, seeing is sacrificed.

The basic steps for performing a vaginal hysterectomy are done in the opposite order of a TAH. The surgeon stands or sits between the legs and inserts a metal retractor in the vagina. Instead of starting from the top of the uterus down to the cervix, she starts from the cervix and works up to the top of the uterus. It's essentially a backwards TAH:

1. Place clamps on the cervix to provide something to pull down on.
2. Cut across the vagina where it meets the cervix.
3. Enter the posterior cul-de-sac, usually by cutting directly behind the uterus with scissors.
4. Clamp, cut, and suture the ligaments on the back of the uterus.
5. Clamp, cut, and suture the tissue and blood vessels along the sides of the cervix until reaching the uterine blood vessels.
6. Enter the anterior cul-de-sac so the bladder can be pushed out of harm's way.
7. Clamp, cut, and suture the uterine vessels.
8. Divide the ligaments on each side.
9. If leaving the ovaries, clamp, cut, and suture the utero-ovarian vessels.

10. If removing the ovaries, isolate the ovarian vessels, then clamp, cut, and suture them.
11. Suture the top of the vagina.

To better understand some of the limitations inherent in the vaginal approach, imagine blow-drying your hair. Usually you do this in a well-lit bathroom in front of a mirror with plenty of room to move your arms and hands. Now imagine blow-drying your hair while sitting inside a dark box with only a small cone of light around your head. You can hardly move your arms over and around your head because you're working in a small space. And you can't see very well because it's dark. Your view and your access are both limited. If you blow-dry your hair daily, you could probably still do a good job because you are so used to the motions.

Now imagine doing something more complicated, like sewing a button to a section of fabric. But you have to hold the needle at the end of an instrument inserted through a piece of PVC pipe—again, with only a small cone of light by which to see. You get the picture. If you've practiced this many times, you can complete the task as long as the conditions remain similar. But what if the pipe gets smaller and the needle won't fit? Or the button is now in a different position than it's supposed to be? Or the pipe is much longer than usual? Or maybe even the holes in the button to pass the needle through don't exist? Under normal circumstances, all will go well. But if there are other factors to consider, another approach will be necessary. The same is true for vaginal surgery. It's a good approach for the uncomplicated patient. But throw in a few curveballs and we need to make a better choice.

These are coarse analogies for the basic limitations of vaginal surgery, but they illustrate why total vaginal hysterectomy (TVH) is not an ideal option for everyone. However, for younger women with a relatively simple problem, it is often the best choice.

Now let's bring in what I call the Surgeon's Logic. What do I think about when deciding which surgical option is best? The two most important keys for the TVH are the need to remove the ovaries/tubes and the blind nature of the operation. When the surgeon performs steps 3 and 6—that is, entering the anterior and posterior cul-de-sac—she doesn't know what she's going to find. Is the anatomy normal or are there adhesions? Remember that the anterior cul-de-sac is the space between the bladder and uterus, and the posterior cul-de-sac is the space between the uterus and rectum. Without a view from the inside first, she must make her best educated guess about what she is likely to find in those two areas. I run through a checklist in my mind of the most important factors that predict a straightforward and successful vaginal hysterectomy. The following list of these factors is not all-inclusive, but it is illustrative.

1. *To take the ovaries or leave the ovaries*: that is the first question. One of the first things I think about when talking with a patient about her surgery is our plan for her ovaries and tubes. Are we going to take them out at the same time or leave them behind? BSO stands for bilateral salpingo-oophorectomy, the medical term for removing the ovaries and tubes. Some surgeons claim they can reliably remove all the ovarian and tubal tissue vaginally, but I disagree. Because the blood supply to this area starts far from the surgeon's reach, it can be very difficult to remove all the tissue completely. In my career, I have seen dozens of women who were told their ovaries were removed vaginally, only to see me years later with a mass growing from one of them. Very commonly, the retained ovary/tube wasn't completely removed during the vaginal surgery years earlier. You can imagine a woman's outrage when she learns she has ovarian cancer, after thinking her ovaries were out years ago. Therefore, if BSO is necessary, the choice for TVH is off the table.

2. The *size* of the patient is also of crucial concern here. If the patient is obese, and especially if she is obese and not had children vaginally, the surgeon's view is limited. That means that if the surgeon encounters bleeding or adhesions, her ability to deal with these adversities can be compromised. In the morbidly obese, she literally may not have instruments long enough to reach the blood vessels of the uterus. The risk of serious bleeding and injury skyrocket, making this approach a poor choice in these cases.

3. *Previous vaginal deliveries*: Having babies makes the uterus easier to remove vaginally. This is an important factor when considering vaginal surgery. The ligaments holding the uterus in place relax during childbirth, allowing it to be pulled closer to the vaginal opening during surgery. If a woman has never given birth vaginally, the TVH can be more challenging.

4. *Previous pelvic surgery* is also a factor in considering whether the TVH is right for you. Scarring in this area means your surgeon may have to separate the colon from the back of the uterus, increasing the risk of a dangerous injury. An especially well-known culprit for scarring between the bladder and the uterus is the cesarean section. When separating the bladder from the uterus and cervix during step 6 of a vaginal hysterectomy, previous cesarean sections increase the risk of injuring the bladder. An even riskier situation is previous intestinal surgery in the pelvis. The lower part of the colon and the top of the rectum sit right behind the uterus and cervix. Scarring in this area means your surgeon has to separate the colon from the uterus, and an injury here can be dangerous. If an injury to the bowel occurs, a serious or even life-threatening infection can occur. For these reasons, most surgeons avoid vaginal surgery when there has been previous pelvic surgery.

5. History of or suspicion of *endometriosis* is a harbinger for adhesions. Nobody knows why some women get this unfortunate condition, but it affects about 15 to 20 percent of all women of reproductive age. Endometriosis can cause scarring in front of and behind the uterus, making blind entry in either area dangerous. In some cases, the disease is so severe that the rectum becomes almost fused to the back wall of the uterus. In this scenario, dissecting the rectum away from the uterus can be challenging enough with open surgery. But entering the pelvis blindly during step 3 of a vaginal hysterectomy is more dangerous and can result in a rectal injury.

6. *Previous infections* of the female organs or previous diverticulitis (an inflammation in the wall of the colon) are portents for

scarring. Pelvic inflammatory disease from previous infections can lead to bands of scar tissue in the pelvis. Adhesions cause organs to be stuck together where they shouldn't be, increasing the risk of injury.

7. Leave no stone unturned: In the case of *cancer* or a suspicion of cancer, a thorough operation is the most important thing on the surgeon's mind. If I can't see, I can't perform a full evaluation of the cancer, potentially missing areas where spread may have occurred. In addition, in many cases of cancer, removal of the ovaries is necessary for cure.

With all these limitations inherent in the vaginal approach to surgery, gynecologists were hungry for a better alternative. What about an operation that would allow a view of the patient's insides *before* entering the pelvis blindly but without the invasiveness of the TAH? Enter the wonderful world of laparoscopy.

LAPAROSCOPICALLY-ASSISTED VAGINAL HYSTERECTOMY (LAVH): SETTING THE TABLE FOR THE FUTURE

With the development of fiber optic technology, the ability to place a small camera inside of the body opened up all kinds of possibilities for MIS. The term laparoscopy means "camera in the abdomen." As a few analogies to understand the medical jargon, arthroscopic surgery signifies putting a camera in a joint, like the knee; thoracoscopy refers to a camera in the chest; and colonoscopy means a camera in the colon. The first laparoscopic appendectomy was performed in 1981, the first laparoscopic gallbladder removal in 1985, and the first *laparoscopically-assisted vaginal hysterectomy* (LAVH) in 1989. With LAVH, the surgeon performs a portion of a hysterectomy laparoscopically, seeing directly into the patient's abdomen. She then completes the remainder vaginally. Not only can the surgeon remove the ovaries and tubes if necessary, but she can also see if the path is clear for entry in front of and behind the uterus—those key steps 3 and 6 we talked about with vaginal hysterectomy. In the early days of laparoscopic hysterectomy, this was the way gynecologists overcame some of the disadvantages we discussed for both the open and vaginal approaches.

The laparoscopic component of an LAVH is usually performed with three or four pea-sized incisions. The surgeon places surgical plastic sleeves in these incisions, which act as a porthole into the body. The camera or different surgical instruments can be passed through these sleeves. Then the abdomen is filled with carbon dioxide gas. This creates space between the organs and the patient's belly wall, creating a work area to safely move the instruments around. The surgeon chooses instruments to accomplish many kinds of tasks such as cutting, dissecting, coagulating, or suctioning. The camera is typically hand-held by an assistant surgeon or operating room technician, moving the camera at the surgeon's instruction to see various parts of the body. When the camera is in the body, the image is magnified on monitors like a TV set, so everyone in the room can see what's going on. The camera is pointed directly at the organs of interest, so the uterus, ovaries, and tubes are magnified on the screen. If the surgeon is thinking about removing the ovaries and tubes, unlike the vaginal approach, she can see them clearly and remove them entirely. Additionally, the areas all around the uterus can be seen. Remember that with the vaginal approach, the space between the bladder and cervix and between the cervix and rectum are entered blindly. In the case of laparoscopy, if the surgeon doesn't like what she sees, she can immediately convert to an open TAH, before an injury occurs.

Typically, at the start of an LAVH, the patient is positioned on the operating room bed with her legs in padded stirrups that can be raised or lowered. Two separate sets of instruments are prepared: one for the laparoscopic portion and the other for the vaginal portion. The remaining steps of the operation follow those of the TAH for the laparoscopic part, and the TVH for the vaginal part. The surgeon divides the ovarian blood supply, the tissue between the side of the uterus and the pelvis called the broad ligament, and then the uterine vessels. She may or may not begin the bladder separation at this point. Then the team—the surgeon, assistant, and surgical technician—steps away from the abdomen and moves between the patient's legs, lifting them up in the air so there is space to stand. The remainder of the hysterectomy is completed vaginally. The uterus is removed through the vagina. The surgeon then reconstructs the top of the vagina with stitches. The team then changes to clean gowns and gloves and refills the abdomen with carbon dioxide gas. The camera is again placed through one of the portholes and the surgical area is inspected to make sure there is no bleeding or sign of injury. Then the small incisions are closed and the operation is complete.

Any technique that avoids a long continuous incision is superior in terms of postoperative pain, shorter recovery, lower overall cost, and less scarring. For the straightforward hysterectomy, the LAVH became a less invasive alternative to open TAH. Studies showed a significant cost savings and improved patient quality of life compared to open surgery. As cameras, monitors, and instrumentation improved, more complicated operations were performed. Skilled laparoscopic surgeons began performing uterine cancer surgery by adding removal of lymph nodes to the hysterectomy. Larger fibroids were removed using a morcellator, a device that cores fibroids like an apple corer until the uterus is small enough to come out through the vagina.

The best thing about LAVH, however, was that it allowed a transition in thinking and training for gynecologic surgeons. Those of us trained in the era before laparoscopy learned open surgery and vaginal surgery very well. Performing the LAVH was an early foray into more advanced laparoscopy while retaining the surgeon's comfort with vaginal surgery to complete the more difficult tasks of dissecting the cervix and closing the vagina. This allowed us to learn to accomplish the steps of a hysterectomy without our hands inside the patient. I also think it created a slow but subtle turn in our mindset to think more personally about how our methods affect the lives of the women on which we operate. If your primary tool for hysterectomy is an open incision, why think about how your incision will affect a patient's body image or her career or her family life? You have nothing better to offer. But if you now have a less invasive approach, it changes how you imagine the operation and how you think about the impact of the operation on every woman you see.

A unique hazard of any laparoscopic surgery is the risk of injury from placing the sleeves. At the beginning of the operation, the laparoscopic sleeves or ports are placed into the abdomen. After the first port, the remaining sleeves are placed once the abdomen has already been distended with the carbon dioxide gas. This allows the surgeon to aim the camera at the spot where the sleeve is coming through the abdominal wall, watching it at all times to avoid injury. However, the first port must go in with limited visualization. Until that port is in, there is no way to expand the abdomen with the gas and thus create a working space for the camera. Injuries to the intestines, bladder, or blood vessels have occurred with sleeve placement and are unique to laparoscopic surgery.

Disadvantages of the LAVH include the extra time and instrumentation required for the vaginal portion of the operation. But most importantly, the inherent drawbacks of the two-dimensional image on the monitor and the limited range of motion of the instruments keep the advantages of minimally invasive surgery out of reach for women with more complex problems.

Your doctor may also be thinking about other considerations when she makes a recommendation for surgery. Soon after laparoscopy became mainstream, surgeons began noticing a physical toll on *themselves*. Reports of neck, shoulder, and elbow injuries in busy laparoscopic surgeons increased, many of which ended careers.[6] In conventional laparoscopy, the surgeon has to hold and manipulate the long instruments with her hands outside the patient's body and create fine movements at the tip of the instrument about a foot and a half away. This is done while watching the monitor screen. As you can imagine, the surgeon often finds herself feeling like a pretzel, contorted and twisted in unnatural positions.

As an alternative to TVH, LAVH became a good option for the straightforward hysterectomy where removal of the ovaries/tubes was planned. However, for a more complicated situation, the LAVH still had many limitations. What if the path is not clear when looking at the inside of the pelvis? What is the fallback plan when the case looks

---

6   Franasiak J, Ko EM, Kidd J, Secord AA, Bell M, Boggess JF, Gehrig PA. "Physical strain and urgent need for ergonomic training among gynecologic oncologists who perform minimally invasive surgery." *Gynecologic Oncology*. 2012 Sep;126(3):437–42.

too complicated for laparoscopy? The contingency plan is always conversion to open TAH. In the Surgeon's Logic, what if I really need to avoid a large incision for a diabetic, obese, or medically ill patient? In the obese patient, both the laparoscopic and vaginal phase of LAVH can be a physical struggle, literally feeling like a fight against a heavy opponent. It is simply much harder to see and reach the important structures in an obese patient. When the abdominal wall is thicker, there is more resistance to the fine movements of laparoscopy, creating much greater fatigue. Unfortunately, the patients who usually benefit the most from laparoscopy are the obese and medically infirm, thus producing a decision dilemma: Do I recommend an MIS approach for my patient when I know how difficult it will be for me physically, even though I know it will benefit her? A busy surgeon may find she can only complete two conventional laparoscopic hysterectomies in a day rather than three or four with another technique. With these time constraints, financial pressures, and patient interests pulling the surgeon in opposite directions, she may recommend the easiest approach for her, rather than the best approach for the patient.

TOTAL LAPAROSCOPIC HYSTERECTOMY (TLH): THE NEXT BEST THING

The question that should be obvious after reading the previous section is "Why not perform the entire procedure laparoscopically?" And the short answer is—because it's harder. More specifically, removing the cervix and stitching the vagina laparoscopically can be quite challenging. These two challenges are precisely the steps performed vaginally in the LAVH. Historically, gynecologists have felt more comfortable tackling these steps of the operation vaginally. This may not intuitively make sense because this portion of a vaginal hysterectomy is done blindly. However, when the vaginal portion is straightforward and the anatomy is normal, finding the natural space between the bladder and cervix is relatively easy to accomplish. The primary tool used to find that space is the surgeon's finger. What could be more natural? Stitching the vaginal cuff is accomplished directly with a stitching instrument in hand. Again, with a straightforward case, the vaginal approach feels more intuitive for the traditional gynecologic surgeon.

Now let's take a closer look at these two laparoscopic challenges outlined previously to better understand the paradigm shift between LAVH and total laparoscopic hysterectomy (TLH). The first challenge is removing the cervix. Before the advent of energy sources like vessel sealing devices, surgeons were still mired in the "Clamp, cut, suture" mantra. Once instruments that seal and divide blood vessels became available, dividing the blood vessels to the cervix became a safe and attainable alternative to the vaginal approach.

The other primary obstacle in TLH involves stitching the top of the vagina after separating it from the cervix. This area needs to be sutured together so it will heal well. Throwing a stitch through tissue requires a turn of the wrist like rotating a doorknob. Imagine trying to open a doorknob with a chopstick. The rotation must come from the shoulder instead of the wrist, but this is not a natural human movement. That is why many surgeons refer to conventional laparoscopy as "straight stick laparoscopy." It's like operating with chopsticks instead of hands. Several modern instruments are available to combat this problem; however, they lack the dexterity and control of directly placing stitches through tissue exactly where they need to go.

Many surgical technology companies have developed great products to overcome some of these disadvantages, allowing gynecologists to become proficient at performing the entire operation laparoscopically. With training and gradual skill development, the TLH became possible. Advantages of this technique over the LAVH include less postoperative pain, a shorter recovery, and lower hospital costs. Avoiding the vaginal portion eliminates the need to place heavy metal retractors in the vagina. This means less pulling and tugging on organs and less trauma to the sensitive skin of the labia and outer vagina. With less pain, women usually go home more quickly from the hospital and return to normal activities faster. No portion of the operation, except the initial placement of the trocar or port, is blind. The entire surgical team sees the patient's insides on the monitor screen. Dissection around the cervix proceeds with direct visualization. And because the operating team only opens one set of instruments, and those same instruments are used for the entire procedure, costs are lower. It just doesn't make financial sense to open a vessel-sealing device for just a few minutes of use, as would be the case for the LAVH, and then switch to standard surgical clamps for the remaining portion of the case. With the TLH, the surgeon can use one device for the entire procedure.

However, the biggest problem with the conventional TLH is that the usual limitations of conventional laparoscopy still apply. The picture is still two-dimensional and the camera hand-held. The surgeon still controls the instruments by hand outside the patient's abdominal cavity, and the instruments only allow limited range of motion. The procedure is still physically taxing for the surgeon due to poor ergonomics.

Comparing LAVH to TLH, the bladder separation is no longer blind. Instead, it's just awkward. In reality, the TLH offers a small incremental improvement over the LAVH, but it's not a game changer. The TLH affords a few advantages over LAVH with respect to post-operative pain and recovery and may be more cost-effective. But the patient who needs MIS the most is still on the outside looking in. The TLH, like the LAVH, favors the straightforward case in relatively thin, otherwise healthy women without cancer.

SUPRACERVICAL HYSTERECTOMY (SH): A DANGEROUS COMPROMISE

Technically, the term supracervical hysterectomy (SH) means "partial hysterectomy" because only a *part* of the uterus is removed. Although many laypeople use the term "partial hysterectomy," I think they mean taking the uterus and leaving the ovaries and tubes. For surgeons, however, the term lacks any specific anatomical meaning. "Partial hysterectomy" doesn't specify which part is removed and which part is retained. Also, anatomically, the ovaries and tubes (adnexae) are considered separate organs from the uterus. When a patient tells me she's had a partial hysterectomy, I can't be sure if she means that the entire uterus was removed but the ovaries were left, the uterus was removed but the cervix was left, or the surgeon removed part of the uterine wall and left the remainder behind. Because of this confusion, the phrase is best avoided. Supracervical hysterectomy is more specific because the term describes what part of the uterus is removed (the uterine body) and what part is left behind (the cervix).

The SH can be performed either abdominally or laparoscopically. In either case, the surgeon cuts the uterus from the cervix, leaving it behind. Why would a doctor want to do this? During the transition from LAVH to TLH, some surgeons began performing a laparoscopic SH. Leaving the cervix in place avoids the difficulties of dissecting the cervix and suturing the vaginal cuff. However, in my opinion, many women are not fully informed about the disadvantages of this approach.

The steps of the laparoscopic supracervical hysterectomy (LSH) are very different from all the other hysterectomies we have reviewed so far. Since the cervix is never separated from the vagina, there is no opening between the pelvic cavity and the outside through which the surgeon can remove the specimen. So how does the uterine tissue come out?

The uterus is an organ made up of a muscular wall and an inner lining. When the uterus is separated from the cervix, all this tissue must be broken up into pieces and removed through the small dime-sized incisions. This is typically accomplished with a tool called a morcellator. This device has a low-speed motor that drives a sharp coring blade that cores the uterine tissue like an apple corer. Each piece is about the diameter of the sleeves, so the tissue cores can be pulled through a sleeve until the entire specimen has been removed.

There are risks associated with this technique. First, a serious injury can occur during the morcellating process. Second, if an undetected cancer is present in any part of the uterus, breaking it up into pieces can spread it throughout the abdomen. Therefore, two key points for safely performing SH include proper training and technique with the morcellator, and ensuring, to the best of the surgeon's ability, the presence of a benign condition.

One clear advantage for SH is that, since the cervix is not removed, the woman can return to intercourse more quickly. When I counsel my patients about sex after hysterectomy, I let them know it's okay to engage in any activity other than intercourse until eight to 10 weeks after surgery. Achieving orgasm soon after surgery is not dangerous. I just want to protect those stitches in the vagina until the area has healed completely. When others tout the faster return to sex as an advantage of LSH, we should clarify that this advantage only applies to intercourse but not specifically to other types of sexual activity. Once the vaginal stitches have healed completely, there are no restrictions to sexual activity after any method of hysterectomy.

It seems that for some time there was a campaign to convince women the SH was better than total hysterectomy. Many articles appeared in women's magazines and shows aired on television extolling the virtues of the cervix, conferring almost magical properties on a structure about the size of the tip of your thumb. People argued that the cervix provides support to the pelvic organs and is important in female orgasm. Neither is true. The support for the pelvic organs comes from the muscles and ligaments of the pelvic floor, a huge web that crosses between the pelvic bones and keeps our organs inside. It's hard to imagine that a structure the size of the tip of your thumb could hold all your intestines inside of you! Sexual pleasure comes primarily from the extensive network of nerves in the labia and clitoris, which connect to the pelvic floor. The waves of sensation during orgasm are actually the pelvic floor muscles contracting in a pleasurable way. There are very few nerves in the cervix itself.

The American College of Obstetrics and Gynecology issued a consensus statement in November 2007, discouraging gynecologists from performing the SH. This opinion was reaffirmed in an updated statement in 2010. The college stated that women should be counseled regarding "the lack of data demonstrating clear benefits over total hysterectomy." It went on to say, "The supracervical approach should not be recommended by the surgeon as a superior technique for hysterectomy for benign disease." Most importantly, it warned that women with any current or recent history of or suspicion for cancer or precancer are "not candidates for a supracervical procedure." Therefore, any woman with an abnormal Pap smear should not have this procedure. Any woman who has abnormal bleeding where there is any possibility of cancer should not have this procedure. Any woman with a history of HPV infection should not have this procedure.

With this statement, the college was stressing that there is no proven advantage to this procedure even when cancer or precancer are not a concern. They also caution that women should be counseled about the potential future need for removal of the cervix. In up to 20 percent of cases, women still have bleeding when the cervix is left in place. Surgically removing a retained cervix, a procedure called a trachelectomy, is quite difficult with a much higher complication rate than hysterectomy. In particular, because of how the body heals after SH, the bladder can become difficult to separate from the cervix, significantly increasing the risk of injury.

The greatest danger with SH occurs when undiagnosed cancer is present. I have had cases referred to me after another doctor performed a SH only to learn in the pathology report that an unknown cancer was present. What a terrible feeling to learn, too late, that bits of cancer were spread around the abdomen. This is a dangerous situation that compromises the survival of the patient. Also, remember that the cervix and uterus are really one continuous structure. If cut apart during surgery and a cancer is present, the cancer cells can spill out. Some of the cancer can also be left behind. It can be very difficult to go back and try to fix this type of situation with additional surgery, radiation, or chemotherapy. Therefore, as an oncologist, I strongly recommend against the SH. In addition, as a gynecologist, I don't endorse any improvement in sexual function or pelvic support with the SH. This compromise is just not worth the risk.

ROBOTIC HYSTERECTOMY:
THE REVOLUTION IS HERE

Robotic surgery was approved by the Food and Drug Administration for gynecologic surgery in April, 2005. Since then, it has rapidly changed the landscape of gynecology from the old-fashioned approaches we just discussed to a complex world of choices and options. It was in September of that same year when I was first introduced to robotic surgery, leading to the epiphany in my surgical practice described in chapter 1. At the time, I was disillusioned with medicine and with the limitations of available surgical techniques. When I discovered what I could do with robotic surgery, I experienced renewed joy and satisfaction with my practice—and I still do today.

Currently, the only available surgical robot is manufactured by Intuitive Surgical Inc. in Sunnyvale, California. Hysterectomy using this system is referred to as *da Vinci* hysterectomy. Although gaining in popularity, most women have never heard of it and certainly don't realize it might be good for them. The vast majority of people don't know what the term "robotic surgery" means. It's time for some enlightenment: robotic surgery is the newest innovation in minimally invasive surgery, and it's the game changer surgeons have been waiting for. This technology gives the proficient surgeon a huge advantage in performing complex operations that previously required a TAH, with all of its disadvantages. With this new technology, there are very few situations where an old-fashioned incision is necessary. No longer is MIS reserved only for easy cases. Now MIS is an option for almost everyone.

There are three physical parts to the *da Vinci* Surgical System. First is the patient cart. This consists of a center post from which extend four interactive arms. This is the portion that actually "docks" to the sleeves inserted into the patient's abdomen. One arm is attached to each sleeve, typically utilizing the center arm to hold the camera. The second part of the system is the vision tower, which houses the light generator and system electronics. Finally, the surgeon console provides an interface between the surgeon's eyes and hands and the instruments attached to the interactive arms. The surgeon sits at this console—comfortable, ready for action, and immersed in a three-dimensional viewing station—and inserts her fingers into the grips. Voila! Any movement she makes, the instruments follow.

How does this technology differ from conventional laparoscopy? First, the binocular camera held by the center arm sends a 3-D, stable, high-definition live video feed to the viewing station. As the surgeon, I maintain control of what I see at all times and can zoom in for a magnified view when necessary. I can move the camera exactly where I need it. The picture is crystal clear, with amazing detail. With the surgical robot, I feel like I'm seeing all the important structures, large and small. Blood vessels pop into view. Nerves are more easily visible. The right tissue planes appear more obvious. With so much additional visual information compared to other techniques, this results in more precision, fewer injuries, and less blood loss. In contrast, with conventional laparoscopy, an assistant hand-holds a one-eyed camera, moving it at the surgeon's instruction. The image is therefore only two-dimensional and shaky. Precision is sacrificed. The surgeon is not in control of what she is seeing because she has to rely on the assistant to aim the camera.

Next, with the *da Vinci* Surgical System, I manipulate all the necessary surgical instruments through a computer interface while sitting at a console next to the patient. These instruments are wristed, meaning they move like a human hand. Conventional tools, also known as "straight stick" laparoscopy instruments, are manipulated by the surgeon's hands just outside the patient's body. Since these instruments have limited motion, the movements can be awkward, resulting in less mobility and precision. This is especially important during stitching, when turning the wrist directs the curve of the needle through tissue. But perhaps even more importantly, with my fingers in the grips of the console, my movements are intuitive and natural. For example, when you reach to pick up a pencil, your index finger and thumb extend together, ready to pinch the pencil between them. On the surgical robot, the motion to reach and grab something, like a blood vessel, is identical. I place my index finger and thumb in the finger grips. Once the system is activated, if I reach and pinch my finger and thumb together, the exact same motion is translated to the surgical instruments inside the patient. When I reach with my right hand, the instrument controlled by my right hand moves precisely where I tell it to go. When I reach toward the side, the instrument moves to the same side. When I reach up, the instrument goes up, and so on.

While operating, I am sitting in a supportive chair, performing the procedure from an ergonomically superior position. For the experienced robotic surgeon, this reduces fatigue and leads to shorter operating times and greater operating room efficiency. Remember that we talked about the physical toll of conventional laparoscopy on the surgeon. With *da Vinci* surgery, surgeons stay fresher throughout the day, improving operating efficiency and prolonging their career. The dilemma faced by minimally invasive surgeons disappears. Now the easiest technique is also the best, both for patients and for surgeons.

The term "robotic surgery" is actually a misnomer. More accurately, the technology of the *da Vinci* Surgical System is best described as computer-assisted surgery. The word robot implies the movements are somehow automated, but this couldn't be further from the truth. I try to avoid the term robotic surgery, because it sounds like I just press a button, go get a cup of coffee, and the surgery happens on its own. I only wish it were that easy. It's simply a tool that connects my movements to the instruments inside the patient's body. When I sit at the surgeon's console, I interface with the system by placing my thumb and index finger into finger grips. The system translates each movement of my hands, in real time, to the instruments through a series of tiny pulleys. I maintain complete control of both the camera and the instruments at all times.

The *da Vinci* Surgical System is available at many hospitals around the world. The technology is expensive, but it is a shared resource utilized by many surgical specialties for a variety of conditions. The first system was introduced in the late 1990s, originally based on technology from the U.S. Department of Defense. Initially, the military was looking for ways to stabilize injured soldiers in the field while the trauma surgeon operated remotely from a secure location. Intuitive Surgical Inc. then developed the system for the operating room.

As with new approaches to almost anything, criticisms of this technology are abundant. The primary critique is its price tag. In the United States, each system costs about $1.6 million. For programs that are busy and create models of efficiency, *da Vinci* surgery has been shown to be more cost effective than other modalities.[7] Mainly, this results from fewer days in the hospital, typically the greatest charge in any hospitalization. These analyses don't even include the costs of home health care, antibiotics, and complications saved

---

7   Geller EJ, Matthews CA. "Impact of robotic operative efficiency on profitability." *American Journal of Obstetric Gynecology*. 2013 Jul;209(1):20.e1–5.

compared to more invasive surgical approaches. As a society, we also save when patients can return to work faster due to a shorter recovery. Also, the system is a shared resource that can be used by many specialties for many different applications, thus improving the cost-to-benefit profile. In my own cases, I choose the ancillary equipment in the room with an eye toward cost containment. Other instruments that are costly, such as stapling devices or electrocautery tools are no longer necessary. We use non-disposable tools for most of the other aspects of the procedure, saving on medical waste expenses as well.

These costs are not charged to the patient. In general, the payment between your insurance company and the hospital is pre-determined based on contracts. The hospital calculates an average cost of these kinds of cases, and they negotiate a payment scale with the insurance company. Many factors determine the overall cost of a hospitalization, but the biggest factor is how long you stay in the hospital. Think of an overnight stay in a hospital as one of the world's most expensive hotel rooms. Each night in your hospital bed ratchets up the costs tremendously. One of the other major costs is the time in the operating room. It is like renting a suite so expensive that you pay by the minute. The more efficiently we use the operating room suite, the more cost-effective the overall hospitalization.

Another expenditure that is hard to quantify is the cost of complications and conversions. Complications can occur during or after any operation. We will discuss these in more detail in chapter 9, but for now, I want to emphasize their contribution to the cost of surgery. A minor complication such as a wound infection can be treated with antibiotics—not a big expense. But a major complication, such as bleeding, can lead to blood transfusions, additional blood work, a prolonged hospitalization, and a longer overall recovery. When a life-threatening complication occurs, such as a blood clot or unrecognized injury, costs become astronomical.

Conversion refers to when the surgeon begins the operation laparoscopically but runs into trouble and has to convert to an open procedure. In these cases, the costs include all those for laparoscopy plus all the costs for open surgery. Not to mention the additional risk and expense of dealing with the complication that led to conversion in the first place. Conversions are expensive and dangerous and need to be minimized.

Finally, equipment costs contribute significantly to the overall expense of your surgery. Certainly, robotic surgery ranks high on the equipment side of the ledger but can make up for it by saving hospital days, complications, and conversions. For the right kinds of cases, this lowers the overall expense to our medical system.[8] Recent publications and media coverage caution against the widespread use of robotic surgery for straightforward hysterectomies due to these high equipment costs.[9][10] I agree we need to better understand which cases benefit most from this technology. Hospitals with formal robotic programs tend to track their costs and outcomes more closely than those that are just jumping on the robotic bandwagon without real oversight and planning. A well-managed program should standardize training for staff, credentialing for its surgeons, and equipment use to minimize costs.

I've also heard criticism that the robot is "dangerous." If you perform a Google search for "robotic hysterectomy," the first websites that come up are attorneys looking to make money from patient complications. These sites claim that somehow the machine can injure patients. That just doesn't make sense. That's like saying cars run over people, so it must be the cars' fault. On rare occasions, a car malfunction leads to an accident. But we all know that most of the time, the operator of the car causes the accident. The same can be said of any surgical tool, whether it be the *da Vinci* robot, a heart-lung machine, or an orthopedic drill. As with any new technology, proper training of surgeons and operating room personnel is key to maintaining patient safety.

---

8   Boggess JF, Gehrig PA, Cantrell L, Shafer A, Mendivil A, Rossi E, Hanna R. "Perioperative outcomes of robotically assisted hysterectomy for benign cases with complex pathology." *American Journal of Obstetric Gynecology.* 2009 Sep;114(3):585–93.

9   Wright JD, Ananth CV, Lewin SN, Burke WM, Lu YS, Neugut AI, Herzog TJ, Hershman DL. "Robotically assisted vs laparoscopic hysterectomy among women with benign gynecologic disease." *JAMA.* 2013 Feb 20;309(7):689–98.

10 "AAGL position statement: Robotic-assisted laparoscopic surgery in benign gynecology." *The Journal of Minimally Invasive Gynecology.* 2013 Jan;20(1):2–9.

Robotic surgery is relatively new, so the medical community is still working out best practices for defining surgeon training, hospital oversight, and operating room team education. This pattern is oh-so-familiar whenever any new technology comes around. Surgeons remember the flurry of lawsuits that occurred when the laparoscopic gallbladder operation first came out. Now, this surgery is the standard of care for gallstones, and known complications of the operation are well described and widely accepted. The same process occurred when the LAVH was first introduced. Many gynecologists said laparoscopic hysterectomy was just a fad. Now laparoscopy is a commonly used technique for many procedures in gynecology.

Other limitations of the current robotic system include limited application to surgery in multiple areas of the body. For example, if the surgeon needs to operate in all areas of the abdomen at once, this technology is limiting. It is a better choice when the procedure involves one defined area, like the pelvis, because the arms all face in one direction. Once the system is set up and docked, moving the whole machine around is cumbersome. In addition, the arms have some limitations to range of motion. Currently, the instruments are wristed, but they have no elbows. In the future, instruments that can bend like elbows would improve range of motion.

The current system also lacks surgeon tactile feedback, the ability of the surgeon to feel the tissues as she works. Certainly, a system with tactile sensation would add an important dimension to the surgeon's interaction with the surgical field. For the most part, this drawback does not affect the quality of the operation in the hands of an experienced surgeon. The surgeon learns to use visual feedback, that is, how the tissues respond to the surgical movements, as a surrogate for tactile feedback. However, in some types of cancer surgery, such as for ovarian cancer, feeling the tissues is crucial to identifying spread of disease. In these cases, I avoid using any method of MIS.

With these limitations in mind, robotic surgery has opened a door that, in the past, was closed to many women. For those who need it most, minimally invasive surgery can save lives. Now, women who would previously have been told to endure the same old-fashioned operation as their mothers and grandmothers can reap the benefits of modern medicine in the hands of modern surgeons. This technology essentially neutralizes the concerns in the high-risk patients we reviewed in the other methods of hysterectomy. For example, an obese woman who has had previous surgery may be able to have a minimally invasive hysterectomy. A cancer patient requiring an extensive removal of lymph nodes may be able to have a minimally invasive hysterectomy. A diabetic with a history of blood clots will have a lower risk of complications with minimally invasive surgery than with open surgery.

Future improvements to robotic technology are close at hand. Reduced port surgery is becoming available, where surgeons can perform the same operation with even fewer incisions than before. Advancements in flexible cameras and bendable instruments allow insertion of multiple devices through one incision, instead of each device going through its own incision. Placing the camera and all the instruments through a single incision means an entire hysterectomy can be done through the belly button.

Image-guided surgery is also on the horizon. For example, use of a special camera detects fluorescence in lymph nodes, guiding removal of only the most important ones and sparing normal tissues. Techniques are under development to detect nerves, blood vessels, and other critical structures with the goal of minimizing trauma and bleeding.

Robotic technology represents the future of surgery. As new developments add to the foundation we have today, computer-assisted surgery will replace and enhance almost everything we currently do in the operating room.

RADICAL HYSTERECTOMY:
FOR CANCER PATIENTS ONLY

Although only accounting for a very small percentage of all hysterectomy types, a basic understanding of the radical hysterectomy provides a framework to understand many important aspects of pelvic surgery, including the revolutionary paradigm shift occurring with robotic surgery. The term radical hysterectomy refers to a very different operation than the total hysterectomy. A radical hysterectomy is performed almost exclusively for cervical cancer and describes a much more extensive operation than the typical hysterectomy. Many women misunderstand this term and believe it signifies a hysterectomy with removal of the ovaries and tubes, but this is not correct. When most people use the term "radical hysterectomy," they are referring to a simple TAH/BSO, the prototypical operation for common female reproductive problems. I think many laypeople mistakenly add the term radical when the ovaries and tubes are included in the hysterectomy. But the radical hysterectomy is only performed by trained gynecologic oncologists for specific cancer treatments, such as early-stage cervical cancer. In the operation, all the lymphatic and vascular tissue around the cervix is removed along with the uterus and cervix. In addition, a portion of the top of the vagina and the surrounding lymph nodes are also removed. Removing all these parts together ensures the best chance of containing the cancer cells during surgery, and therefore, the best chance of cure. In order to take out this extra tissue, a much more extensive dissection around the bladder and ureters is required. Removing the lymph nodes is done to check for spread that would indicate a more aggressive cancer. If the lymph nodes are involved, radiation and chemotherapy are usually necessary to control additional spread.

In my own subspecialty of gynecologic oncology, proficiency in this operation is the cornerstone of our surgical training. The skills required to successfully perform the radical hysterectomy translate into the expertise of an experienced pelvic surgeon. The real key is safely and precisely dissecting the ureters away from the surrounding tissue. This requires good visualization, precision, and dexterity. For decades, this operation was performed through large open incisions. Women generally spent about five days in the hospital and then another six to eight weeks at home recovering. Before the era of robotics, a few gynecologic oncologists tried performing this operation with conventional laparoscopy. The results were not very good. The operation took a lot longer to complete, and the complication rate was higher. However, when all went well, the patients did recover much faster. This benefit encouraged most gynecologic oncologists to look for a better way to accomplish the operation with a minimally invasive approach, but very few felt comfortable adopting conventional laparoscopy in its current state at the time.

With the advent of robotic surgery, the open radical hysterectomy is a thing of the past. Now this extensive cancer operation is performed through several dime-sized incisions requiring only an overnight stay in the hospital. About 40 percent of gynecologic oncologists in the United States are robotically active, and many in our field around the world have published their results with the robotic technique, demonstrating low complication rates and few conversions.[11] [12] [13]

Many of you may remember the saying, "We've come a long way, baby." I certainly feel that way when I think about the modern hysterectomy compared to the hysterectomy of the past. With all the techniques available today, how do you and your surgeon come to a decision for you? We are no longer in the age of your mother's hysterectomy; now we are in the age of *your* hysterectomy. Let's go there next.

11 Cantrell LA, Mendivil A, Gehrig PA, Boggess JF. "Survival outcomes for women undergoing type III robotic radical hysterectomy for cervical cancer: a 3-year experience." *Gynecologic Oncology*. 2010 May;117(2):260–5.

12 Boggess JF, Gehrig PA, Cantrell L, Shafer A, Ridgway M, Skinner EN, Fowler WC. "A comparative study of 3 surgical methods for hysterectomy with staging for endometrial cancer: robotic assistance, laparoscopy, laparotomy." *American Journal of Obstetric Gynecology*. 2008 Oct;199(4):360.e1–9.

13 Mendivil A, Holloway RW, Boggess JF. "Emergence of robotic assisted surgery in gynecologic oncology: American perspective." *Gynecologic Oncology*. 2009 Aug;114 (2 Suppl):S24–31.

Chapter 8

THE SURGEON'S LOGIC AT WORK:
NOW IT'S YOUR HYSTERECTOMY

Now that you understand the evolution of the modern hysterectomy, let's delve into the Surgeon's Logic as she thinks about you when you come to her office. What's your hysterectomy story going to be? What kind of surgery will be done—open, vaginal, laparoscopic, or robotic? Will your hysterectomy be different from your mother's? Your grandmother's? What are your concerns and fears?

The title of this book, *Not Your Mother's Hysterectomy*, reflects the advances in modern medicine compared to past generations. When patients come to see me for consultation, their expectations are often based on their mother or their sister or their friend's hysterectomy. They frequently ask questions like, "Well, my sister had her hysterectomy in such and such way, so why am I different?" To this question, I say, "*Everyone* is different." No two cases are the same. We are all unique individuals with individual histories and individual problems that bring us to the doctor in the first place. For example, fibroids and abnormal bleeding are very common, but every woman who carries those fibroids is different. In surgery, the nitty-gritty details are important. Your *symptoms* may be the same as your friend's, but your surgery may be very different. For example, maybe your friend had a vaginal hysterectomy for fibroids, but your uterus is twice the size of hers. Or, maybe you had two cesarean sections, while your friend did not. These differences matter and can dramatically change the way your surgery should be performed.

It's natural for a woman to compare herself to family members who had a hysterectomy. Your mother's hysterectomy was likely an old-fashioned TAH. For you, even something as simple as your age could have a large impact on your surgical approach. For these reasons, my first piece of advice is: don't compare yourself to anyone else. Your situation must be taken individually and approached with a unique strategy.

Some of the issues that bear upon this strategy are based on important medical considerations, and others are based upon your own feelings and wishes. When I apply my Surgeon's Logic to your case, I must consider the medical issues first. Your feelings and desires are very important, but medical decisions should first rest on what's best for your health. For example, you may want to avoid a large incision, but if you have a huge mass with extensive adhesions, I may not be able to avoid one without putting your life in jeopardy. I understand your feelings, but I also must do what's safe. My job is to explain this to you, to translate my Surgeon's Logic to you.

The primary considerations we will cover in this section include the pros and cons of the different methods of hysterectomy and whether or not to remove the ovaries and tubes at the same time. As you read, remember that the term hysterectomy refers only to removing the uterus and cervix. From a medical standpoint, removal of the ovaries and tubes is considered a separate operation. The proper term for this procedure is a *BSO*: bilateral (meaning both sides) salpingo (meaning removal of the fallopian tubes) oophorectomy (meaning removal of the ovaries).

Let's talk about your ovaries first. The decision regarding BSO can affect you in several important ways: fertility, menopause, probability of future cancer, and risk of future surgery. During your reproductive years, your ovaries produce hormones and carry your eggs. Removing the ovaries prior to natural menopause, therefore, puts you into a surgical menopause and renders you unable to get pregnant. If you are already past childbearing age, then loss of fertility from a hysterectomy is not a concern for you. However, if you need a hysterectomy but were hoping for children in the future, this decision can be a harrowing one. Many premenopausal women seek alternatives to hysterectomy for just this reason. In general, if you've come to the doctor for a problem so severe that you would sacrifice your childbearing potential to correct it, you're already ready for a hysterectomy. However, if you are seeking alternatives to hysterectomy, please discuss these in detail with your doctor. Those treatments are outside the intended scope of this book, but I encourage a thorough dialogue with your doctor to explore all your options. Some patients who need a hysterectomy, even those with cancer, are able to preserve their ovaries safely. For example, the treatment of early cervix cancer in young women does not require removing the ovaries in most cases. These cancers don't typically spread to the ovaries. I follow several young patients who had a radical hysterectomy for cervical cancer but were able to keep their ovaries. Later, they were able to have their own children using a surrogate. Options exist, so discuss your feelings with your doctor.

Unfortunately, that is *not* the case for uterine or ovarian cancers. Because these cancers can involve both ovaries and tubes, they should be removed in most cases. Leaving them in place can lead to a higher risk of cancer recurrence and ultimately death from the cancer.

Unlike uterine and ovarian cancers, treatment for non-gynecologic cancers doesn't typically include BSO. However, if radiation is required for treatment, it will destroy the eggs and the hormone production in the ovaries, leading to premature menopause in younger women. Radiation can also affect the uterine lining, making it unreceptive to future pregnancy. Fortunately, in young women, advanced reproductive technologies can allow retrieval and storage of eggs prior to starting radiation. Hormonal treatments can then be given after the cancer treatment is complete to support a pregnancy with the stored eggs. For these women, hope for a family can be a guiding light through grueling cancer treatment.

After loss of fertility, the next common concern among women needing hysterectomy is their fear of menopause. Let's face it, none of us look forward to "the change." And if you're already there, you may be living with these changes every day. But menopause is different for every woman. Some experience terrible hot flashes; others very few. Some women experience a change in sleep habits or mood swings. Others are most bothered by vaginal dryness or decrease in sex drive. No matter how it affects you, it's usually something we hope to put off as long as possible.

Someone once said to me, "we shouldn't call it meno-pause, we should call it meno-STOP." It's not a pause; it's permanent. The term menopause simply describes the phase in your life when your ovaries stop producing hormones. Without these hormones, menstrual cycles stop permanently, and you can no longer get pregnant. The uterus itself produces no hormones; its only function is to carry a pregnancy. During your reproductive years, the uterus responds to the hormonal cycles of your ovaries, resulting in a menstrual cycle. When those hormonal cycles cease, so do your periods. The fallopian tubes do not make hormones either; only the ovaries produce hormones. These hormones include estrogens (there is more than one type), progesterone, and various androgens like testosterone. The average age of menopause in the United States is 51. Therefore, once in their early fifties, women don't produce these hormones anymore, and *that* is menopause.

When making the decision about how to approach your surgery, if you are already 50 or older, it is generally recommended to remove the ovaries and tubes during your hysterectomy. The primary advantage of removing them is to reduce your risk of ovarian cancer. Additionally, many women will develop benign masses in the ovaries or tubes later in life that will require additional surgery. Research shows that about 10 percent of all women who retain their ovaries after a hysterectomy will need another operation in the future to remove a mass.[14] Taking them out at the time of hysterectomy spares you from that future risk of additional surgery. For some women, that risk is significant. For example, if future surgery is no small undertaking due to obesity or a history of multiple previous operations, it may be best to take out the ovaries today to prevent the need for additional surgery tomorrow.

Many postmenopausal women are confused when we discuss removing the ovaries during hysterectomy. They frequently ask, "Will I need to take hormones after this surgery?" These women are already in menopause. I explain to them that once their ovaries are no longer producing hormones, removing them shouldn't change things. It would be like removing your appendix. It has no function, so if it's removed, you'll notice no difference. The same is true with the ovaries in menopause. If they're not functioning now, then removing them doesn't change that. Therefore, it you're not taking hormones now, nothing should change after hysterectomy/BSO.

However, if you need a hysterectomy and have *not* gone through menopause yet, then your ovaries are still functioning and still producing hormones. In that case, you and your surgeon will need to

---

14 Casiano, Elizabeth R. MD, MS; Trabuco, Emanuel C. MD, MS; Bharucha, Adil E. MBBS, MD; Weaver, Amy L. MS; Schleck, Cathy D. BS; Melton, L. Joseph III MD; Gebhart, John B. MD, MS. "Risk of oophorectomy after hysterectomy." *Obstetrics & Gynecology*. 2013 May;121(5):1069–74.

make a decision about whether to take them out at the time of your hysterectomy. Consider these important factors:

1. If you have a cancer that could spread to the ovaries/tubes, they probably need to come out.

2. Your risk of future abdominal surgery. If you are overweight or have had extensive previous abdominal or pelvic surgeries, you are at increased risk for a surgical complication. You and your doctor must consider that future risk against your desire to preserve fertility and avoid menopause.

3. Your family history of cancer. If you are at increased risk for breast or ovarian cancer, you and your doctor may elect to remove your ovaries along with your uterus to lower your cancer risk. Consider genetic testing first to better understand your risk.

4. Benign conditions that affect your ovaries. For example, endometriosis can persist if the ovaries are left. Endometriotic tissue can be stimulated by ovarian hormones and may cause problems after hysterectomy without BSO. In severe cases, BSO may be required. In addition, BSO may be the only option for alleviating chronic, painful ovarian cysts.

A recent study of over 30,000 women showed that women who have their ovaries removed before the age of 50 and don't take hormones have a significantly higher chance of dying at a younger age from all causes except ovarian cancer. They were much more likely to die younger from cardiovascular disease like stroke or heart attack and all other types of cancer.[15] Discuss these statistics with your doctor when making your decision about your own ovaries.

---

15 Parker, William H. MD; Feskanich, Diane ScD; Broder, Michael S. MD, MSHS; Chang, Eunice PhD; Shoupe, Donna MD; Farquhar, Cynthia M. MD, MPH; Berek, Jonathan S. MD, MMS; Manson, JoAnn E. MD, DrPH. "Long-term mortality associated with oophorectomy compared with ovarian conservation in the nurses' health study." *Obstetrics & Gynecology.* 2013 Apr;121(4):709–16.

Next, let's look at some women who face different types of hysterectomies. When presented with the choice, why do most women prefer the minimally invasive method? Simply put, who wants to be cut open if you don't have to? That's why the laparoscopic hysterectomy is now replacing the open hysterectomy for many women.

Shonna is a 48-year-old woman with fibroids and abnormal bleeding. When her periods start, she can't work because the cramping is so severe. She is anemic due to excessive blood loss and has gained weight because she doesn't have the energy to exercise. Her uterus is only slightly enlarged, and she weighs about 180 pounds. She wants her ovaries removed at the time of the hysterectomy because her mother and grandmother both had breast cancer at a young age. The ovaries make estrogen, so by removing them she will enter a surgically induced menopause. In her case, this is purposeful: removing her ovaries may lower her risk of getting breast cancer by decreasing hormonal stimulation to the breast tissue. She is a perfect candidate for a TLH/BSO.

Another good candidate for TLH/BSO is Kristy, a 52-year-old smoker with recurrent precancer of her cervix. Her Pap smears have been abnormal as long as she can remember, and her doctor is concerned about her risk of cervical cancer. Cervical cancer is a smoking-related cancer just like lung cancer. She is 120 pounds and has never had surgery before. She is already menopausal and wants her ovaries removed.

In these relatively straightforward cases, the surgeon has several choices of which method to recommend for TLH. A conventional laparoscopic approach by an experienced surgeon would be an excellent choice. Others, like me, would recommend the *da Vinci* hysterectomy. Some surgeons might perform these laparoscopic hysterectomies with single-site instruments, minimizing the number of scars. The real advantage between robotic techniques and all others becomes apparent when the cases become more complex.

For Vicki, the thought of another open incision was terrifying. She was a 300-pound diabetic with very large fibroids and life-threatening bleeding. She had already been transfused with 10 units of blood over the last two years. One year ago, another surgeon operated on her and took out a large ovarian cyst but wouldn't do her hysterectomy due to her obesity. She came to me with a two-foot long scar from that operation, which took several months to heal after a serious infection. Her uterus was larger than it was the year before, about the size of a five-month pregnancy, due to the fibroids.

The challenges with her case included her obesity, large uterine size, and adhesions from previous surgery. For a case like this, before the availability of robotics, she would have needed another large incision, with all the attendant risks and healing difficulties. However, I was able to perform the operation through five dime-sized incisions, and she went home on the second postoperative day. Her pain was minimal and her bleeding cured.

As you can see from these examples, certain factors are especially critical in surgical decision making. These decision points guide much of the Surgeon's Logic. When you ask the question "Which method of hysterectomy is right for me?" the answer is, "It depends."

"It depends on what?" you may ask. Well, practically everything, but some decision points are real deal breakers. Let's go through these in detail; however, please do not consider my words to constitute actual medical advice. It's always best to discuss all your concerns with your doctor and come up with a treatment plan together.

In the following table, I have summarized the most important decision points discussed throughout the book. I have listed the common methods of hysterectomy, what advantages each offers, the types of incisions required, the average hospital stay, and the expected recovery time. I also added a comments section covering specific considerations. In terms of the relative pain score, I based this purely on my own experience and not on any scientific study comparing all the techniques. In my own practice, having performed all the types of hysterectomy except the SH, I have found that open incisions cause the most pain, so I rated them highest on the pain scale.

Let's go through the table in detail and look at each method in turn. First is the TAH or open hysterectomy. This operation is best reserved for complex cancer cases or barriers to laparoscopic sleeve placement. What are barriers to sleeve placement? Remember that to perform any MIS, the first step requires placing sleeves in the

Method of Hysterectomy	Best For	Incisions	Average Hospital Stay (days)	Return to Normal Activities (weeks)	Pain (1=least, 6=most)	Considerations
TAH	Ovarian cancer Metastatic cancer Barriers to sleeve placement Need for abdominal exploration	1 large incision, vertical or horizontal	3–5	6–8	6	Highest risk for infection, blood clots, scarring, and metabolic, heart, and lung stress Tactile feedback
TVH	Keeping ovaries No previous surgery Normal weight Prolapse	None	1	4–6	1–2	Risk of bladder or rectal injury Less visualization Can perform concomitant vaginal reconstructive surgery
LAVH	No advantages	3–4 pea- or dime-sized	1	4–6	3	Less OR efficiency Risk of port placement Post-op CO_2 pain
Open SH	Cesarean or post-delivery hysterectomy	1 large incision, vertical or horizontal	3	6–8	6	Must exclude cancer Bleeding can persist Quicker return to intercourse
LSH	Best avoided	3–4 pea-sized and 1 dime-sized	1	3–4	3	Must exclude cancer Bleeding can persist Morcellator size contributes to pain Quicker return to intercourse Risk of port placement Post-op CO_2 pain
cTLH	Uterine fibroids Abnormal bleeding Cervical or uterine precancer Small pelvic masses No previous surgery Not obese Minimal previous surgery	3–5, pea- or dime-sized; or a single 1 inch incision	1	3	1–3	Single-site possible with only 1 incision Risk of port placement Post-op CO_2 pain Surgeon ergonomics inferior to robotics
rTLH	Pelvic masses Uterine fibroids Large uterus Previous surgery Endometriosis Pelvic prolapse Obesity Uterine cancer Cervical cancer	3–5, pea- or dime-sized; or a single 1 inch incision	1	3	1–3	Low risk of complications Can perform concomitant prolapse repair Surgeon ergonomics Most surgical dexterity Risk of port placement Post-op CO_2 pain Single-site possible with only 1 incision in less complex cases

TAH   Total Abdominal Hysterectomy
TVH   Total Vaginal Hysterectomy
LAVH Laparoscopically-Assisted Vaginal Hyst.
SH   Supracervical Hysterectomy

LSH   Laparoscopic Supracervical Hyst.
cTLH Conventional Total Laparoscopic Hyst.
rTLH Robotic Total Laparoscopic Hyst.

abdomen through which the camera and instruments pass. When patients have extensive scarring from previous surgery, the intestines may be plastered to the abdominal wall. Placing a device into such an area could injure them. Additionally, adhesions can block the view of the camera or block the instruments from entering the abdominal cavity. Large masses can also be a barrier to sleeve placement, especially when a large mass is present in a petite patient. A large mass can literally take up all of the available space in the abdomen, leaving no place to insert a camera or any other necessary instruments.

Why are complex cancer cases often performed through large open incisions? Because open incisions afford the opportunity for abdominal exploration and access to all the abdominal organs. A fundamental principle of cancer surgery involves removal of the primary tumor and assessment of spread to other areas based upon risk. In the case of ovarian cancer, the entire abdominal cavity is at high risk of spread. Therefore, as I write this, my biggest concern with any minimally invasive approach to ovarian cancer is the possibility of missing malignant tumor areas because of the inability of the surgeon to put her hands in the abdomen and feel the surfaces of all the organs. When dealing with ovarian cancer, the surgeon must evaluate the entire abdomen and pelvis for possible spread of disease. If a spot is missed, it could affect the patient's survival. This recommendation may change as new technologies emerge that allow tactile feedback and adequate visualization with scopes.

Other gynecologic cancers, such as cervical or endometrial, are less likely to spread throughout the abdominal cavity. These cancers typically spread to lymph nodes, which can be satisfactorily evaluated with minimally invasive techniques. However, if high risk factors for abdominal spread are identified prior to surgery, then open exploration may also be indicated. For example, if a woman's uterine cancer has spread to her intestines, I need both tactile sensation and access to the whole abdominal cavity to remove the cancer and to check for signs of spread.

Finally, in terms of risks of surgery, any operation carries a risk of infection, bleeding, injury, blood clots, wound healing problems, hospital errors, and anesthesia, heart, and lung complications. The TAH carries the highest risk for most of these concerns: highest risk of infection due to wound size, the highest risk of blood clots due to immobilization, the highest risk of scarring from tissue manipulation, the highest risk of hospital errors from a longer length of stay, and the highest stress to the heart and lungs in the recovery period.

The vaginal hysterectomy (TVH) is a good choice when the uterus is not excessively large, the ovaries are not an issue, adhesions are not expected, and the patient is not obese. It is an excellent choice for prolapse, because many procedures for repairing weakness of the pelvic floor or a dropped bladder are also performed vaginally. Doing all the procedures at the same time with the same access makes sense. The patient has no abdominal scars from a vaginal hysterectomy, and the hospital stay is usually just overnight.

All laparoscopic techniques carry the unique risks of injury from placement of the sleeves (ports) and the possibility of postoperative pain from the use of carbon dioxide gas (CO_2). With modern techniques for laparoscopy, I don't see any advantage to the laparoscopically-assisted vaginal hysterectomy (LAVH). The operation encompasses both the unique risks of laparoscopy and the additional limitations of the vaginal approach. In addition, LAVH results in additional operating room costs and the inherent inefficiencies of two set-ups.

As I discussed in the section on supracervical hysterectomy, I worry about the risks associated with this operation. The primary advantage is a quicker return to intercourse. Occasionally, an open SH is necessary after cesarean section or a vaginal delivery when massive hemorrhage occurs. In this setting, identifying the cervix can be difficult, especially if the patient has gone through labor and the cervix is thinned. When the goal is saving the patient's life from bleeding, spending the extra time dissecting out the cervix may not be in the patient's best interests.

Another consideration with leaving the cervix is that some women will still bleed. Going back and removing a retained cervix is a difficult operation with a much higher risk of urinary injury compared to performing a total hysterectomy from the start. Because the uterus isn't there to pull on for traction, the cervix is harder to separate from the bladder and ureters.

I place the LSH higher on the pain scale because a morcellator is required in every case to remove the uterine tissue. Morcellating devices are 15 millimeters in diameter and therefore larger than the typical 5–12 mm sleeves used for other laparoscopic methods. The larger the incision, the greater the pain. In addition, manipulating the morcellator can cause more trauma at the incision site, contributing to postoperative pain.

One caveat with my pain scale should be noted here: some conventional total laparoscopic hysterectomy (cTLH) and robotic total laparoscopic hysterectomy (rTLH) cases also require a morcellator if the uterus is too large to fit out through the vagina intact. In these cases, postoperative pain would be equivalent to the LSH, accounting for the range in the pain scale for these methods.

The cTLH is useful for many simple, benign hysterectomies. The word total, in total laparoscopic hysterectomy, means the operation is totally laparoscopic (no vaginal portion) *and* a total hysterectomy is performed (the uterus and cervix are both removed). Shortcomings of this approach become apparent as the complexity of the case rises. In addition, this method suffers from the worst surgeon ergonomics of all available techniques.

Naturally, what many women want to know is: "Am I a candidate for robotic surgery?" Certainly, rTLH offers all the advantages of MIS, even for complex cases. I find most women gravitate toward this method because they intuitively grasp the advantages of better vision and wristed instruments. The key to successfully completing a hysterectomy robotically is the ability to place the camera and the sleeves with enough space to see and to work. If you had previous surgery that caused extensive adhesions, they could obscure the view during camera or port insertion. With that said, in my experience, this rarely occurs. I have successfully completed robotic surgery on women who have had multiple previous cesarean sections, previous intestinal surgery, previous endometriosis surgery, previous colon cancer surgery, previous hernia surgery, previous liver and kidney transplants, and even previous abdominal defect repair at birth. Patients often come to see me pessimistic about their chances of avoiding another incision, especially if they had a bad experience in the past.

In most cases, I am pleasantly surprised at what can be accomplished with better technology and some ingenuity.

Let's talk about some examples of cases that I could *not* complete robotically without conversion to open surgery. Take the case of Ruth, a 76-year-old woman who had her entire colon removed due to ulcerative colitis and colon cancer. She now lives with a permanent ileostomy (a bag for her stool) on the right side of her abdomen. She was referred to me after being diagnosed with uterine cancer. Often, removal of the entire colon will result in extensive, widespread abdominal adhesions. We had a long discussion before the surgery, where I shared my concerns about the likelihood of conversion. She wanted to give it a try, but, despite our best efforts, we were unable to place the ports for her surgery. We completed her TAH/BSO uneventfully, and she has recovered well.

I was hoping to complete Sybil's surgery robotically. She is a 66-year-old obese diabetic with uterine cancer. However, as we started the hysterectomy, I saw that her cancer had already spread beyond her uterus into the surrounding pelvic tissues. We had to convert to an open procedure, and I ended up removing her uterus, ovaries, and tubes, along with the affected colon.

A few years ago, I operated on a 92-year-old woman with uterine cancer who had surgery so long ago they closed her belly with metal wire. Her body had such a strong reaction to the wire that the adhesions were fierce, and we had to convert to open surgery.

The key to a successful and safe outcome with any hysterectomy is to choose wisely before you enter the operating room. For this reason, discuss your medical history, your concerns, and your wishes with your surgeon in the office so the best choice is clear. That way, both you and your surgeon can set realistic expectations for your surgery and your recovery. Your hysterectomy story starts with this consultation. How it ends depends on how things go in the operating room and how your recovery proceeds from the moment you wake up. Let's explore the postoperative experience further in the next chapter.

Chapter 9

TOWARD A HAPPY ENDING:
RECOVERING YOU

In early 2013, Joyce Reed came to see me for a second opinion. Joyce was a real estate agent who spoke loudly, with deprecating humor and a broad smile. I asked her what brought her in to see me, and I could tell she needed to get something off her chest.

"My last doctor cancelled my surgery after I spent five hours in the hospital waiting for my hysterectomy," she said bluntly. She was scheduled for a TAH because her fibroids were "too big." "I couldn't afford to lie in a hospital bed for three or four days and be out from work for eight weeks in the first place. Now, it's even more delayed! I was so angry!" Joyce said. "Why did that doctor make me wait all that time just to send me home?"

Whoa! Let's back up and hear the whole story.

Another doctor had diagnosed uterine fibroids several years ago, Joyce told me, but they weren't causing her any problems then and she was told to just keep an eye on them. Over the past two years, they grew much, much bigger. She was exhausted all the time and bled terribly. When she bent over to pick up the dog, she felt like she would pass out. She was self-employed and the only breadwinner for her household. On top of that, she took care of her disabled husband who had suffered from a stroke. Even though she knew things were getting worse, the bottom line was, she was scared. She was scared of surgery. Scared of being put to sleep. Scared of not being able to get up by herself. Scared of being dependent. Where would the money come from while she was out? But the bleeding was sucking the life out of her.

Finally, her girlfriend convinced her to get something done. Joyce, her friend Cathy, and Cathy's sister had been the closest of friends. Cathy's sister had recently died of cancer, and it was Cathy's pleas that ultimately made her face her hysterectomy. "I don't want to lose you, too," she cried to Joyce.

Joyce's gynecologist examined her and ordered a scan. Her fibroids were huge, the size of a woman six months pregnant. This doctor didn't do major surgery herself, and wisely referred Joyce to a gynecologic oncologist for her operation. Joyce had heard about robotic surgery from one of her clients who marveled at being in the hospital for only a day and back to work in a week. Joyce wondered if this was possible for her, too. The gynecologist was skeptical, but she wouldn't be the one doing the surgery.

The gynecologic oncologist told Joyce that robotic surgery was not an option for her. It just couldn't be done. Joyce resigned herself to this reality and showed up for her operation reluctant but ready. It turned out she had an abnormal EKG that hadn't been addressed prior to the day of the operation. After fasting, getting an IV, and waiting for five hours, she was sent home, understandably irritated and frustrated.

Joyce immediately went to her office and got on the Internet. She had heard my name before and looked me up to get a second opinion.

After examining Joyce that day, I could see why the other doctors were skeptical. Her uterus was almost up to her rib cage. But I felt there was a reasonable chance I could be successful robotically. In my earlier years with robotic surgery, I would not have attempted to do this robotically, but by then I had enough experience with challenging cases that I felt confident in this approach. After listening to her home situation, I understood how important it was to her to recover as fast as possible. I gave her a 50/50 chance of success that the surgery could be completely done robotically. I described how I would put the laparoscopic camera in to see if it was possible. If not, we would proceed the old-fashioned way with a faster surgery but a much longer cut. If robotic, it would take several hours to break up all those fibroids, but she would only have four dime-sized incisions.

"What do I have to lose?" Joyce asked her girlfriend, who had accompanied her to the office visit. "There's a 50/50 chance. Let's try it," Joyce concluded.

In the operating room, we planned the position of the incisions based on the massive size of her uterus.

"This looks like the uterus that ate Cleveland," my assistant said in wonder as I started the operation.

But as we carefully worked, the dissection went beautifully. It took less than an hour to separate the uterus from the surrounding structures. Then the real work began—breaking the uterus up into small enough pieces to remove through the small incisions. We used the device called a morcellator, specifically designed for this purpose.

It took over two hours of continuous work to get those fibroids out. My hands were numb, but I was so proud.

We took photos of the uterine pieces on a scale because we had achieved a record for the largest uterus yet removed laparoscopically in Las Vegas. I went out to the waiting room to see Cathy and showed her the pictures.

"I just knew when we met you that everything would be all right," she said in relief. "I am so glad that other surgery got cancelled. I guess everything happens for a reason."

When Joyce opened her eyes in the recovery room, she couldn't feel anything yet. The first thing she asked was, "Where is a clock?" If it went fast, then it was the Big Cut. But she saw four hours had elapsed, and she was elated. Her fear was gone. Her hope had become a reality.

• • •

When you think about it, you are asleep during your operation. You put your life in your doctor's hands when the mask goes over your face. It's when you wake up that you begin to measure the success of your surgery. You will judge the entire experience based on how you feel the first day, the first week, the first month, and maybe even years later. Setting realistic expectations for your recovery is an important part of the process.

Naturally, most people worry about how much pain they will feel when they wake up. But what about when you get home? Who will take care of you? When will you see the doctor? What were the results of the surgery? When can you go back to work? When can you resume normal activities? What will sex feel like afterward? These are important questions to think about before surgery, and you should discuss them with your doctor or her staff in the pre-operative period.

The typical stages of a surgical recovery include the immediate postoperative period, the first day, the first week, the first month, and the rest of your life. Within each stage, there are milestones to monitor your progress. These milestones depend on your type of hysterectomy.

There are essentially three postoperative scenarios in gynecology: the minimally invasive hysterectomy (whether for benign or malignant indications), the open benign hysterectomy, and the open cancer hysterectomy. The expectations for all three differ significantly.

A minimally invasive hysterectomy, done with a TVH, LAVH, cTLH or rTLH, usually requires an overnight hospital stay, although some surgeons only keep patients for a few hours of observation before discharge.

In the second scenario, the simple TAH for general gynecologic conditions is performed through one continuous incision, either vertical or horizontal. This incision must be large enough to admit a surgical retractor and all the instruments that will be necessary to accomplish the hysterectomy, including the surgeon's hands. A woman undergoing a TAH will require a longer stay than MIS and, on average, may stay in the hospital three days.

In contrast, a TAH, done as part of an extensive cancer operation or other complex procedure, is probably contributing much less to the overall recovery than the other components of the surgery. For example, when a woman with ovarian cancer has a TAH along with removal of other organs such as a portion of her intestine, she may need a week or more in the hospital. When a hysterectomy is one small part of a bigger operation, the recovery is difficult to predict and addressed on a case-by-case basis. Therefore, I will focus minimally on this scenario due to its variability. No matter which type of hysterectomy you need, discuss your own case in detail with your doctor.

Many aspects of each stage of recovery are shared among all types of hysterectomies. I will point out the differences for the common concerns most women raise with me in my practice.

THE FIRST FEW HOURS

In the immediate postoperative period, you will go to a surgical recovery unit called the recovery room. Most people wake up there, and a few stay on a breathing machine until they are more stable. This is where Joyce Reed first woke up looking for the clock. She didn't feel sore at all until she moved around a little or had to cough. She was amazed she didn't feel more "out of it."

Obviously, Joyce's case went beautifully, but not everyone sails through recovery so easily. The riskiest period after surgery is in these first few hours. For this reason, the hospital staff monitors vital signs frequently. Some patients also experience nausea. Expect to have an intravenous line infusing fluids, oxygen given by nose or face mask, a catheter in your bladder, and some discomfort. Many patients feel cold after surgery, and warming you up is an important part of your nursing care. Many hospitals cover patients in warm blankets or wrap them in a plastic bubble circulated with hot air.

All laparoscopic operations and most open procedures require general anesthesia. With general anesthesia, your breathing muscles are paralyzed during the operation. This allows the best control over your vital functions during surgery, such as gas exchange and circulation. Side effects include the well-known grogginess and nausea typical of the first few hours after an operation.

Most of my patients receive epidural anesthesia in addition to general anesthesia. One of the advantages of an epidural during surgery is the ability to inject a long-acting pain medicine that minimizes pain for the first twelve hours. The epidural also minimizes bowel activity during surgery, improving overall safety. Less pain results in avoidance of intravenous narcotics. The use of IV narcotics, such as morphine, has been shown to delay recovery and prolong hospital stay. They slow bowel motility, increase nausea, and result in a sluggish patient who doesn't want to walk. By utilizing the long-term pain relief of the epidural in combination with the rapid return of appetite with MIS, patients can immediately transition to oral pain medicine, thus avoiding the intravenous route.

THE FIRST DAY

In the first day after her hysterectomy, Joyce Reed was amazed at how good she felt. She had some discomfort, meaning a little dull soreness, but no sharp pain. She was able to get up on her own, and her appetite was back. She remembers looking over the menu and actually feeling hungry for hospital food. She was able to urinate on her own and felt independent.

At that point in her recovery, Joyce was in a surgical ward. After demonstrating stable vital signs, alertness, and adequate pain control, expect to transition to a similar unit within a few hours after surgery. In the next twelve to twenty-four hours, the primary goals of the staff include assessing your status, assisting you in regaining mobility, controlling pain, monitoring intake, and preparing you for discharge. To assess your condition in this period, the staff will continue monitoring your vital signs, though not as frequently as in the recovery room. Every four hours is the standard. Your fluid intake and urine output are also measured and recorded.

Typically, your blood is drawn early in the morning the day after surgery. Common tests include a complete blood count and basic metabolic panel, which help identify postoperative infection, anemia, or electrolyte abnormalities. Measurement of kidney function also helps evaluate fluid status and check for signs of a urinary injury. Expect to be awakened for a blood draw—these tests are extremely important.

Most people worry about being laid up for a long time after surgery and relying on others for every little thing. One of the keys to regaining mobility is early ambulation: sitting up in bed, dangling your legs, sitting in a chair, walking around the room, and eventually walking in the hallways are critical for avoiding common and serious complications of most surgical procedures. Moving around decreases the risk of blood clots, improves breathing, lowers the risk for pneumonia, maintains stamina, and assists in return of bowel function and appetite.

Pain control is one of the obvious distinctions between MIS and open approaches in this early postoperative period. There is a big difference between taking a few pain pills and being on an intravenous narcotic pump. Avoiding pain is a basic human instinct, and minimizing it is one of the great game changers of the newer surgical techniques. Ask your mother or other family member who had a hysterectomy a generation or two ago, and pain may be the first memory that comes to mind.

One of the keys to rapid recovery is avoiding intravenous narcotics. For patients with open incisions, our surgical team recommends leaving the epidural in place for a few days. This helps with pain, decreasing but usually not eliminating the need for intravenous narcotics. Patients feel more awake and alert, with less nausea. However, large incisions hurt, and it's impossible to keep a patient completely pain-free after a big operation.

Women with open incisions dread getting in and out of bed after surgery because it hurts. Instead of trying to sit up, it's easier to roll onto your side and push yourself up to sitting with your arms. Then swing your legs over the side of the bed. When getting back into bed, do just the opposite. You may need help initially getting your legs into the bed. Then lie on your side and roll onto your back. A hospital-style bed that tilts up at the head is very helpful.

Coughing can also be painful. Hold a small pillow against your stomach when you cough to minimize the pain in the incision.

The first postoperative day for an MIS patient is busy. The bladder catheter is removed early in the morning and you get up with assistance from the hospital staff. Patients are usually given a full breakfast, anticipating a rapid return of appetite. After your surgeon or surgeon representative (physician assistant or nurse practitioner) makes rounds, the discharge process begins. This involves paperwork and education to ensure proper documentation of your progress and a safe trip home.

Gas pain after surgery is common for all types of abdominal operations. This comes from the effect of anesthesia on the intestines as well as any manipulation of the bowels during an operation. Once you start to pass gas, the pain improves significantly. Moving around stimulates the gas to pass more quickly.

Another primary difference between MIS and open surgery on postoperative day one is diet. Patients with open surgery can usually only tolerate clear liquids. Because the bowels have been manipulated much more during the surgery, forcing food may result in nausea and vomiting. By contrast, most patients with MIS can eat just a few hours after surgery.

In addition, patients with open surgery can move and walk much less than with MIS. Increased pain also results in shallower breathing, increasing the risk for pneumonia and fever. An important tool to lower these risks is the incentive spirometer, a breathing device that all patients should be given immediately after surgery. The apparatus encourages deep breathing by sucking in on the mouthpiece. The incentive spirometer measures your effort, so you have something to shoot for.

One side effect unique to laparoscopic surgery is shoulder pain. This can occur when carbon dioxide gas, used to create space between your abdominal wall and your abdominal organs, gets trapped under your diaphragm. The nerves that give sensation to the diaphragm are shared with the nerves to the shoulder, so the brain interprets the trapped gas as shoulder pain. This usually goes away on its own within twenty-four hours and is not dangerous.

Preparation for discharge begins almost immediately upon admission to the surgical ward. A hospital bed is one of the most expensive night's sleep you'll ever have (or not have, because they wake you up a lot). Hospitals are under close scrutiny to keep lengths of stay short and control costs. For most cases, the hospital is paid a fixed amount no matter how long you stay. There is a tight balance between ensuring your safety and maintaining profitability, and thus sustainability, for hospital systems. I am not suggesting you should be concerned about the hospital's bottom line, but the longer you stay, the more at risk you are for hospital-acquired infections, hospital errors, and other complications.

To meet criteria for discharge, you should be able to urinate, be free of fever or nausea, demonstrate the ability to tolerate food, and achieve adequate pain control. These milestones signify you no longer need the acute care setting of a hospital. As long as you don't need acute care, you are much safer recovering in your own home than in a hospital.

THE FIRST WEEK

On her first morning home, Joyce was able to fix her disabled husband breakfast. She had bought a whole freezer full of frozen dinners, thinking she wouldn't be able to cook for herself or her husband. She never ate them. She had also bought a pile of magazines to read but never looked at them. She was back in the office on her fifth day. Worried she was unfairly pushing herself, her staff asked, "What are you doing here?" But she reassured them. "I'm fine," she said. She drove herself to her first office visit with me, and stopped along the way to buy me flowers and chocolate. When I saw her walk in with a vase of flowers, a box of chocolates, and a great big smile on her face, I stopped what I was doing and soaked it in. I knew this surgery had made a big difference in her life, and it showed.

Usually within a week or two of hospital discharge, you will see your physician for your first postoperative checkup. This office visit is to evaluate your progress, look for any signs of a complication, review the surgical findings, and answer questions. Your surgeon will want to know about your pain level, your activity, your diet, and your bowel and urinary function. Any concerns about these issues should be shared with your doctor. Your surgeon will want to check your incision(s) and give you feedback on how they look. This is the time to discuss strategies to minimize scarring. Many patients want to use a product to improve the appearance of the scar(s). I advise most patients that once their sutures dissolve, it's safe to use vitamin E oil, or a product like Mederma® to minimize scarring.

Review of your pathology report is critical. I give all my patients a copy of this report for their records. Keep your copy in a safe place for future reference. The pathology report is the written examination of the organs that were removed your body. Your final diagnosis comes from this report. From the pathology findings and the observations of your surgeon during the operation, your doctor should be able to explain the *cause* of your symptoms. In other words, talk to your doctor about the why behind your hysterectomy. Make sure you completely understand what she says.

In your first week home, you should monitor several aspects of your progress. This list is not meant to be exhaustive, because no one can predict every possible complication. Call your doctor with any concerns. Don't wait until the postoperative visit to report a problem that you think might be serious. The first thing to look for is fever. Take your temperature twice a day. A temperature higher than 100.3 is considered a fever and could be a sign of infection.

Monitor your bowel habits. Abdominal surgery frequently causes constipation, as do pain pills with narcotics. It's important to take a laxative or stool softener to keep your bowels moving. Built-up stool is a common cause of postoperative pain and bloating. Profuse, watery, and frequent diarrhea after any hospitalization can be a sign of a serious, hospital-acquired infection and should be reported to your doctor.

Bladder catheterization is necessary during and immediately after hysterectomy but increases the risk of urinary tract infection (UTI). If you have urinary frequency, blood in your urine, burning with urination, or pain with urination, these could be signs of a UTI.

Part of any hysterectomy involves suturing the top of the vagina where the cervix was separated. The stitches in the vagina take some time to heal, and a small amount of bleeding and/or drainage is common. Heavy vaginal bleeding, an amount similar to a period, is obviously a cause for concern and should be reported immediately. Foul-smelling drainage can be a sign of infection and should also be discussed with your doctor. Leakage of urine or stool from the vagina can signify a rare but very serious injury and should be reported immediately.

Swelling in one leg can be a sign of a potentially serious complication called a blood clot. The affected leg may hurt, but often a blood clot is painless. The danger occurs if the blood clot travels from the leg to other organs like the lungs. A blood clot in the lung

TECHNICAL DETOUR: BONUS READING MATERIAL

A quality pathology report should not be taken for granted. For a straightforward case, most pathologists are capable of providing an accurate diagnosis. However, when a case is unusual or rare, the expertise of a specialist may be necessary. Just as in other areas of medicine, there are specialists in gynecologic pathology. A general pathologist may send a case to a specialist for review if she needs outside consultation. If you feel uncomfortable with any aspect of your pathology report, you can also request an outside review.

In addition, appropriate specimen processing is not standardized, and good communication between the surgeon and the pathologist is necessary to achieve the most accurate results. For example, if a patient has risk-reducing surgery for BRCA mutation, the pathologist will not necessarily know the patient is a mutation carrier unless the surgeon informs her. This is extremely important because the ovaries and tubes are processed differently for BRCA patients.

is called a pulmonary embolus and can be deadly. The risk of blood clots generally continues for about thirty days after surgery. Being active and drinking plenty of water can help alleviate the risk. Avoid flying in a plane or sitting for a long time in a car during this time. Some patients with a high risk for clots are sent home on a blood thinner to lower their risk. All patients should receive this blood thinner while in the hospital.

Swelling in both legs can occur if the body is not properly processing the fluids given during and after surgery. Kidney problems or a weak heart are often key contributors. If you already take a diuretic (water pill), make sure your doctor instructs you on when to resume your medicine after discharge.

Shortness of breath can also be a sign of a pulmonary embolus, heart failure, pneumonia, or even a heart attack. This symptom should be taken seriously and immediately reported to your doctor.

A fundamental principle of healing your surgical wound involves keeping it clean and dry. Your surgical wound(s) should be cleaned according to your doctor's instructions. With MIS, I close the small incisions with self-dissolving suture and then seal the skin with skin glue. This allows my patients to shower right away and clean the incision with soap and water. A scab will usually form and takes about a week to flake off. The skin sutures dissolve in about three to four weeks.

Consider the case of Nancy, a 45-year-old woman with a pelvic mass. At the time of her surgery, an ovarian cancer was identified. She underwent a TAH/BSO, removal of the omentum, and removal of pelvic and abdominal lymph nodes. The surgeon failed to communicate his expectations to the pathologist, assuming she knew how to process all the specimens. The technician only sampled two small areas of her omentum, which was the size of a hand towel. These two samples did not show cancer. Was Nancy's omentum clear of cancer or did the lab fail to identify spread because the technician didn't process enough samples to find it? I saw this patient for the first time when she came in for a second opinion a month after her operation. I carefully read the pathology report and called the pathologist and asked him to process more of the omentum, but it was too late. She had already disposed of all the tissue. Now the patient is left never knowing the true stage of her cancer and having to decide between fewer or more treatments with chemotherapy due to the uncertainty. Inadequate specimen sampling could have been avoided by a direct conversation between the surgeon and the pathologist.

Avoid lifting anything heavier than about 10 pounds for the first week after surgery. This could put undo strain on the abdominal incisions and on the vaginal incision. Wounds can open up from too much stress until they are properly healed. For open surgery, I recommend patients avoid lifting for at least a month or longer, depending on the size of the incision.

After surgery, it's important to eat a good balanced diet with fiber, fluids, and protein. Regaining stamina starts with walking, increasing the distance a little bit more each week. For more strenuous exercise, my rule of thumb is this: if it doesn't hurt, it's okay to do it. Use your common sense. If something hurts this week, wait to try it again next week.

If your ovaries were removed during your surgery and you were pre- or perimenopausal, you may feel the effects right away. Hot flashes, mood swings, and difficulty sleeping are the most common menopausal symptoms. Discuss these feelings with your doctor. Treatment is individualized for each woman and beyond the scope of this book.

THE FIRST MONTH

It took about two weeks for Joyce to stop looking at her bed sheets every morning for bleeding. It just hadn't sunk in yet that she would never bleed again. By the third week, she was overwhelmed with new energy. She started doing all the things she had avoided for so long. She enjoyed walking her dog, but she had been so tired before that it was a chore. Now, she actually looked forward to cleaning her house because she now had so much energy. She felt free. She felt empowered. She felt like a new woman. She got her happy ending.

In the weeks after surgery, returning to work will probably dominate your concerns. Your type of work affects your recovery from surgery, so discuss your work situation with your doctor. Patients with sedentary professions can generally return more quickly than patients with physical jobs. The primary obstacles to work are pain and fatigue. For MIS, the incisions are so small that returning too quickly is unlikely to cause any medical endangerment. However, doing too much too soon is painful and exhausting. You are unlikely to perform well if you are not ready. In contrast, patients with open surgery who perform manual labor could tear stitches or cause a hernia if they perform their normal duties too soon.

Returning to activities also depends on the type of work environment and the level of activity to which you are accustomed. A marathon runner who manages a restaurant is going to need more time than an accountant who doesn't exercise. Light exercise such as walking is usually safe. More strenuous exercise or housework should be avoided until your doctor gives the okay.

Resuming intercourse should also await the green light from your doctor. After the uterus and cervix are separated from the top of the vagina during hysterectomy, this area is closed with dissolving sutures. We call the top of the vagina after hysterectomy the vaginal cuff. It's important to make sure the stitches have completely dissolved and the vaginal cuff is completely healed before putting anything in the vagina. There is nothing wrong with having an orgasm by engaging in other types of sexual activity. Only vaginal penetration must be avoided. I tell patients that when you find yourself interested in sex, that's a signal from your body that you are probably ready.

THE REST OF YOUR LIFE

Long-term effects of surgery are rarely examined in medical studies. But I get questions from patients all the time about what changes they can expect over the long run. One obvious change includes never having a period again (a welcome break for many women). Other not so obvious ones include change in bowel habits, effect on future colonoscopy, chronic pelvic pain, need for pelvic exams, and sex drive.

Some women report a change in their bowel habits after a hysterectomy. Presumably, their uterus was removed because there was something wrong with it. If the uterus was large, it may have been interfering with bowel movements and a hysterectomy may improve things. Other women report constipation after surgery. The most likely cause for this would be formation of scar tissue after surgery. Because of the trauma of surgery, people can form bands of adhesions that are abnormal connections of scar tissue between nearby structures. The more traumatic an operation, the greater the likelihood of scar formation. Excessive bleeding and infection also increase internal scarring. If adhesions occur to the intestines, colon, or rectum, they can affect bowel function and contribute to constipation.

Adhesions after hysterectomy have also contributed to incomplete colonoscopy.[16] Scarring around the colon or rectum can impede a physician from safely passing a colonoscope, leading to an incomplete attempt at the procedure. Unless followed up appropriately by an x-ray test for cancer, some colon and rectal cancers could be missed.

These adhesions can also cause pain. For some women, chronic pelvic pain after surgery can be debilitating. Any pelvic surgery, including appendectomy, removal of an ovarian cyst, removal of an ovary or tube, bladder surgery, intestinal procedures, and others can be the culprit.

It's surprising how many women stop going to the gynecologist after their hysterectomy.

"Everything has been removed, so why do I need a pelvic exam?" you may ask.

I remind you that not everything has been removed; you still have a vulva, a vagina, a urethra, an anus, and a rectum. Probably no doctor other than your gynecologist is going to check these areas for disease, so yes, you still need a regular pelvic exam.

A healthy sex life is an important part of return to normalcy for many women. Removing the uterus, in and of itself, should not affect your sex drive or enjoyment of sex for you or your partner. If your ovaries needed to come out, too, then you may feel a difference, especially if you were premenopausal. The hormones made by the ovaries have a strong impact on sex drive and the intensity of sexual feelings. Hormones are also important for vaginal lubrication. Vaginal dryness is a common complaint among menopausal women and can make sex more painful. Removal of the ovaries at the time of hysterectomy should not have much effect on a woman who is already well

---

16   Church, J., Garrett KA. "History of hysterectomy: a significant problem for colonoscopists that is not present in patients who have had a sigmoid colectomy." *Diseases of the Colon and Rectum*. 2010 Jul;53(7):1055–60.

into the menopause. But for younger women, these changes should be discussed with your doctor so you are prepared to deal with them.

Finally, I want to say a few words about hormone replacement therapy (HRT). This is a very controversial topic, and new information becomes available regularly that updates our knowledge about the subject. HRT has been covered extensively in other books, but the most important resource for you is your own doctor. You should discuss the pros and cons with her so you can make an educated decision. I would like to note that in some situations, taking HRT should be avoided. First, severe endometriosis can recur from hormonal stimulation, so many of these patients will need to find alternatives to HRT. Also, HRT can increase the risk of blood clots in some women. Finally, some cancers are hormone dependent, and HRT could contribute to a cancer recurrence. In these cases, HRT is best avoided.

Chapter 10

PARTING THOUGHTS

My personal crisis led to a transformation in my practice of medicine that ultimately made me a better doctor, and, I believe, a better person. It's ironic to think that some robot helped me connect more deeply with my patients, but for me, that was the case. I feel that writing this book about my journey has helped me distill my years of training and experience into something palatable to women looking for answers in a time of need. The writing process has taught me new ways to better communicate with my patients on an everyday basis.

As you synthesize the information in this book, I hope you will take away a few key points. First, your body is your own. We pay attention to the food and water we put in our bodies. We know about the importance of regular physical exercise, stress management, and a good night's sleep. But what about the quality of medical care we receive? Although this book is about the common experience many women have with hysterectomy, the concepts can be applied to any interaction with the health care system. Participating in your own medical care is just another way of taking care of your body.

Listen to your gut. When someone treats you with respect and compassion, you know it. The same should be true with your health care providers. Although being sick can be terrifying, anxiety about your doctor's qualifications or ability should not compound the problem. You should walk out of your doctor's office feeling confident with your care, not uneasy and ignored.

Finally, if you need a hysterectomy, or any operation, be prepared. Keep a folder with all your medical records so you and your doctors will always have access to your medical history. Compile a list of all your medications, allergies, drug reactions, surgeries, and medical issues. Know what to expect when recovering from surgery and ask questions about anything you don't understand or about which you want clarification.

Medical care continues to evolve, and robotic surgery is one stone on this long path of progress. In the future, better techniques will assuredly come along. Many of the operations we do now will soon be performed entirely through one tiny incision or incision-free through a natural body orifice like the mouth or vagina. It is also possible that one day my dream of "thinking the operation" could become the new modern reality. An advance like that would certainly warrant a rewrite of this book. Until then . . .

—*Dr. Lynn Kowalski*

GLOSSARY OF TERMS

ANATOMICAL TERMS

Adnexae	Referring to the ovary and tube together.
Anterior cul-de-sac	Anterior means in front of, so this is the lowest area of the front of the pelvis, between the bladder and the uterus.
Bladder	The pelvic organ that stores urine until it's convenient to urinate.
Bladder flap	The portion of the bladder that sits on top of the cervix and vagina. The bladder flap is dissected away from the cervix during a hysterectomy to avoid injuring the bladder.
Broad ligament	A thin membrane of tissue connecting the uterus, ovaries, and tubes to the pelvic side wall.
Cervix	The neck or bottom of the uterus. This is the area that dilates during childbirth.
Fallopian tubes	The tubular structures that connect directly to the uterus and provide a passageway for the egg released during ovulation to the uterine cavity.
Ovaries	The small, whitish-colored organs that contain all the eggs a woman has at birth. They also produce most of a woman's sex hormones.
Pelvic floor	A complex of muscles and ligaments at the bottom of the pelvis that provide support for the internal organs.
Peritoneal cavity	The space within the abdominal cavity that holds all the abdominal organs. This space does NOT include the bones, nerves, or major blood vessels in the trunk; these structures are outside of the peritoneal cavity.
Posterior cul-de-sac	Posterior means in back of, so this is the lowest area of the back of the pelvis, between the uterus and rectum.
Rectum	Lower part of intestine that stores stool.
Ureters	Tubes that propel urine from kidneys to bladder.
Uterus	The muscular organ in the middle of the pelvis where pregnancies develop. Also known as the "womb." In most cases, when we say uterus, we are referring to both the uterus and cervix as one organ.
Vaginal cuff	The top of the vagina after the cervix has been removed. Instead of the cervix at the end of the vagina, a smooth pouch exists in its place.

SURGICAL TERMS

BSO	Bilateral salpingo-oophorectomy. Removal of both ovaries and tubes.
da Vinci Surgical System	The three-part system used to perform computer-assisted or "robotic surgery." The system consists of the vision tower, the surgeon console, and the patient cart with four interactive arms.
Endometrial ablation	The lining of the uterus is destroyed by either heat or other chemical reaction as a means of treating abnormal uterine bleeding.
Hysterectomy	A general term for removal of the uterus.
Laparoscopy	MIS in the abdomen and/or pelvis.
Laparotomy	Surgery in the abdominal-pelvic cavity done through an open incision. The surgeon's hands perform the surgery directly in the patient's body with direct visualization.
LAVH	Laparoscopically-assisted vaginal hysterectomy; a portion of the surgery is done laparoscopically and the remainder done vaginally.
Midline incision	A vertical or "up and down" incision on the abdomen.
MIS	Minimally invasive surgery; this refers to surgery done through small keyhole incisions in the patient's body.
Morcellate	The process of breaking up an enlarged uterus or solid mass into pieces so it can be removed through a smaller opening. Often a mechanical device is used to accomplish this.
Myomectomy	Removal of one or more fibroids from the uterus without removing the uterus itself. This is done when the fibroids are causing or contributing to infertility.
Pfannenstiel incision	Also known as a "bikini cut." This is an incision made across the lower abdomen, usually just at about the pubic hairline.
Radical hysterectomy	A special type of extensive hysterectomy done for cervical cancer. Extra tissue around the cervix, the upper part of the vagina, and the pelvic lymph nodes are removed.
Radiofrequency ablation	Radio waves are conducted to a fibroid to destroy it without moving the uterus.
Robotic surgery	A commonly used term for surgery using the *da Vinci* Surgical System. The term "computer-assisted" is a more accurate description of the interface between the surgeon and the instruments.
SH	Supracervical hysterectomy; removing the uterine body and leaving the cervix. Technically, this describes the "partial hysterectomy." Although many lay people use the term "partial hysterectomy," this phrase is best avoided because it lacks any true anatomical meaning to convey what actually happened in the operating room. When a patient tells me she's had a partial hysterectomy, I can't be sure if she means that the entire uterus was removed but the ovaries were left, the uterus was removed but the cervix was left, or the surgeon removed part of the uterus and left the remainder behind. The latter scenario is almost never the case, but strictly speaking, that is what the term "partial hysterectomy" implies.

Simple hysterectomy	A typical hysterectomy for many benign conditions.
Surgical menopause	The loss of estrogen and other hormones due to surgical removal of both ovaries. When menopause is caused by removal of the ovaries, hormonal changes are abrupt and often more intense at the beginning of the process. Removing one ovary should not lead to surgical menopause. Even a portion of one ovary will continue to make hormones.
TAH	Total abdominal hysterectomy; removal of the uterus and cervix through an abdominal incision while visualizing the organs directly.
TLH	Total laparoscopic hysterectomy; a hysterectomy performed entirely through small incisions using a fiber optic camera for visualization. The specimen comes out through the vagina after it has been dissected from the surrounding structures.
Total hysterectomy	Specifying removal of the entire uterus and cervix as opposed to partial hysterectomy.
Trocar	The sleeve that surgeons use in laparoscopy to pass the camera and instruments through. Synonyms include port or cannula.
TVH	Total vaginal hysterectomy; removal of the uterus and cervix while operating through the vagina.
USO	Unilateral salpingo-oophorectomy. Removal of one ovary and its attached fallopian tube.
Uterine artery embolization	Blocking the blood vessel to a large fibroid. This is done by a radiologist who threads a catheter through the blood vessels in the groin into the main vessel giving blood supply to a fibroid. A small plug or seal is placed in the vessel to stop the blood from reaching the fibroid.

FEMALE CONDITIONS

Adenomyosis	A benign condition similar to fibroids that causes an overgrowth of the muscles and glands of the uterus. It can also lead to pain and abnormal bleeding.
BRCA	A group of breast cancer genes. There are currently two known genes in the BRCA family, BRCA1 and BRCA2, which produce proteins in the cells of our bodies that help repair our DNA when there is an error during DNA replication. Some families have a mistake or mutation in this gene that a parent can pass on to their children, increasing their risk of breast, ovarian, and other cancers.
Cervical cancer	Cancer of the bottom of the uterus. The cervix is the area evaluated by Pap smears.
DUB	Dysfunctional uterine bleeding. This refers to abnormal bleeding in a menstruating, premenopausal woman. The bleeding can be abnormal in frequency or amount or both.

Endometriosis	A benign but sometimes debilitating condition that is believed to come from a reaction to retrograde menstruation. When women menstruate, some of the blood backs up into their pelvic cavity. In some women, the body attacks this blood as a foreign substance, causing inflammation, pain, and sometimes infertility.
HPV	Human papilloma virus.
Menopause	The cessation of menstrual periods that occurs with loss of estrogen production by the ovaries. Once this occurs, the condition is permanent. The natural process is slow and gradual.
Menstrual cycle	The regular coordinated bleeding that occurs in a premenopausal woman signifying communication between the brain, the ovaries, and the uterine lining.
Ovarian cancer	Cancer of the lining or the substance of the ovary. These cancers can also involve the fallopian tube.
Perimenopausal bleeding	Bleeding that is abnormal in timing or amount during the transition to menopause. Usually this refers to a woman's late forties and early fifties. This is the most difficult type of bleeding to evaluate because it can be a normal part of the body's adjustment to less estrogen and therefore less coordination of the body's release of hormones. Or, it can signify serious pathology such as precancer or cancer, as the prevalence of these conditions is on the rise in this age group. It is always best to discuss abnormal bleeding with your doctor.
Postmenopausal bleeding	*Any* bleeding in a woman who has already stopped menstruating is abnormal and should be immediately evaluated by a physician.
Precancer	When the cells lining an organ become abnormal but have not yet become cancer. Precancers are not invasive, therefore they cannot spread to other tissues. If not treated, precancer can become cancer over time.
Primary peritoneal cancer	A cancer that looks and behaves identically to ovarian cancer but starts in the cells lining the abdominal cavity instead of the cells lining the ovary.
Uterine cancer	Usually referring to cancer of the uterine lining. This term can also refer to cancer of the uterine muscle. Pap smears are not designed to detect uterine cancer.
Uterine fibroids	Benign tumors or growths in the uterine muscle. These are the most common reason women need a hysterectomy because of the pain and abnormal bleeding they can cause.

RESOURCES

For access to supplementary bonus content please visit *http://www. DrLDK.com* and use the following password: DrLDK. There you can download these lists with more detail and see updated information to help you through your hysterectomy.

MY HYSTERECTOMY PREP LIST
IMPORTANT FACTS ABOUT ME

1. Age
2. Previous pregnancies and deliveries
3. Current symptoms
   a. Time frame
   b. Severity
   c. Previous treatments
   d. Any factors that make you better or worse
4. Desire for future children
5. Medical problems
6. All previous surgeries, including dates, indications, type of incision, pathology
7. List of any medication allergies
8. All current medications, including prescription or over-the-counter, with dosages
9. Smoking and drug/alcohol history
10. Family history, especially of cancer. Include age at diagnosis of any family member with cancer, type of cancer, and current status.
11. Feelings about menopause
12. Feelings about possible future surgery
13. Feelings about reconstructive surgery
14. History of anesthetic complications in you or your family
15. History of problems taking any particular pain medications
16. Type of work
17. Type of exercise
18. Any household or social situations that would affect surgery or surgical recovery

WHAT TO BRING TO MY DOCTOR'S APPOINTMENT

1. My "Important Facts About Me" list
2. Copies of imaging study reports including ultrasounds, CT scans, MRI scans, and PET scans
3. Actual films from these studies, typically copied onto a CD by the radiology facility
4. Pap smear reports
5. Any relevant biopsy reports
6. Any relevant operative and pathology reports from previous surgeries
7. Treatment summaries of previous therapies for anything related to your current condition, such as previous chemotherapy

QUESTIONS FOR MY SURGEON

1. Are you board certified in Ob/Gyn?
2. If you are seeing a gynecologic oncologist: Are you board certified in gynecologic oncology?
3. Where did you train?
4. How many surgeries do you perform, on average, per week and per month?
5. Do you perform MIS? (If the answer is no, I recommend finding another doctor.)
6. Do you perform robotic surgery? If yes, how many robotic cases have you performed?
7. On average, how many robotic cases do you perform per week, per month, and per year?
8. If MIS is under consideration, what is your rate of conversion to open surgery?
9. What is my diagnosis?
10. What surgery are you recommending?
11. What do you recommend about my ovaries?
12. Am I a candidate for robotic surgery?
13. What are the potential complications of my surgery?
14. Will you be the one actually doing my surgery?

WEB RESOURCES FOR FURTHER READING

For more information about hysterectomies and supplemental material to this book, please visit my website at *http://www.DrLDK.com* or *http://www.notyourmothershysterectomy.com*. There, you can find downloadable versions of "My Hysterectomy Prep List" and "Questions for My Surgeon."

You can also visit my YouTube channel, DoctorKTV, at *http://www.youtube.com/user/DoctorKTV* for videos of robotic surgery and patient education seminars.

For more information about my Las Vegas practice, please visit *http://www.nvscc.com*.

For general information regarding women's health issues, see *http://www.acog.org/For_Patients* and/or *http://health.nih.gov*.

For information about specific gynecologic cancers, visit *https://www.sgo.org*. Go to the bottom of the home page and click on the cancer of interest to you.

For more information about hysterectomies, visit *http://www.nlm.nih.gov/medlineplus/hysterectomy.html*.

For more information about CA-125 for screening of ovarian cancer, see *http://www.cancer.gov/cancertopics/pdq/screening/ovarian/health professional*.

For more information about endometriosis, visit *http://en.wikipedia.org/wiki/Endometriosis#Formation_of_ectopic_endometrium*.

For more information about BRCA, visit *http://www.facingourrisk.org*.

For more information about nonsurgical treatment for fibroids, visit *http://www.medicinenet.com/uterine_fibroids/article.htm*.

ABOUT DR. LYNN KOWALSKI

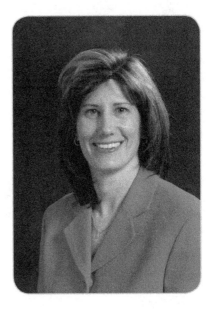

Dr. Lynn Kowalski is a gynecologic oncologist practicing in Las Vegas, Nevada, since 1998. She has performed thousands of hysterectomies with a special interest in minimally invasive surgery. With her extensive training and experience in the many approaches to hysterectomy, she is uniquely qualified to counsel patients about their options.

Dr. Kowalski approaches her practice of gynecologic oncology with compassion and expertise. She has also participated in the training of many young gynecologic surgeons to build a foundation for future leaders in the field. For more information about her practice, visit *http://www.nvscc.com.*

To watch videos of Dr. Kowalski's actual robotic procedures and/or to view educational seminars, visit her YouTube channel at *http://www.youtube.com/user/DoctorKTV.* To view more interactive content from *Not Your Mother's Hysterectomy*, visit *http://www.notyourmothers hysterectomy.com.*

CPSIA information can be obtained
at www.ICGtesting.com
Printed in the USA
BVHW05s1711170618
519089BV00007B/64/P